Aortic Diseases

Editor

FERNANDO FLEISCHMAN

CARDIOLOGY CLINICS

www.cardiology.theclinics.com

Consulting Editors
JORDAN M. PRUTKIN
DAVID M. SHAVELLE
TERRENCE D. WELCH
AUDREY H. WU

August 2017 • Volume 35 • Number 3

ELSEVIER

1600 John F. Kennedy Boulevard • Suite 1800 • Philadelphia, Pennsylvania, 19103-2899

http://www.theclinics.com

CARDIOLOGY CLINICS Volume 35, Number 3
August 2017 ISSN 0733-8651, ISBN-13: 978-0-323-53225-9

Editor: Stacy Eastman
Developmental Editor: Alison Swety

Cardiology Clinics (ISSN 0733-8651) is published quarterly by Elsevier Inc., 360 Park Avenue South, New York, NY 10010-1710. Months of issue are February, May, August, and November. Business and Editorial Offices: 1600 John F. Kennedy Blvd., Ste. 1800, Philadelphia, PA 19103-2899. Customer Service Office: 3251 Riverport Lane, Maryland Heights, MO 63043. Periodicals post-age paid at New York, NY and additional mailing offices. Subscription prices are $326.00 per year for US individuals, $604.00 per year for US institutions, $100.00 per year for US students and residents, $398.00 per year for Canadian individuals, $758.00 per year for Canadian institutions, $464.00 per year for international individuals, $758.00 per year for international institutions and $220.00 per year for Canadian and international students/residents. To receive student/resident rate, orders must be accompanied by name of affiliated institution, data of term, and the *signature* of program/residency coordinator on institution letterhead. Orders will be billed at individual rate until proof of status is received. Foreign air speed delivery is included in all *Clinics* subscription prices. All prices are subject to change without notice. **POSTMASTER:** Send address changes to *Cardiology Clinics*, Elsevier Health Sciences Division, Subscription Customer Service, 3251 Riverport Lane, Maryland Heights, MO 63043. **Customer Service: 1-800-654-2452 (U.S. and Canada); 314-447-8871 (outside U.S. and Canada). Fax: 314-447-8029. E-mail: journalscustomerservice-usa@ elsevier.com (for print support); journalsonlinesupport-usa@elsevier.com (for online support).**

Reprints. For copies of 100 or more, of articles in this publication, please contact the Commercial Reprints Department, Elsevier Inc., 360 Park Avenue South, New York, NY 10010-1710. Tel.: 212-633-3874; Fax: 212-633-3820; E-mail: reprints@elsevier.com.

Cardiology Clinics is also published in Spanish by McGraw-Hill Interamericana Editores S. A., P.O. Box 5-237, 06500, Mexico D. F., Mexico; in Portuguese by Reichmann and Alfonso Editores Rio de Janeiro, Brazil; and in Greek by Dimitrios P. Lagos, 8 Pondon Street, GR115-28 Ilissia, Greece.

Cardiology Clinics is covered in *MEDLINE/PubMed (Index Medicus), Excerpta Medica, The Cumulative Index to Nursing and Allied Health Literature* (CINAHL).

Contributors

FRANCIS J. CAPUTO, MD
Assistant Professor, Division of Vascular
Surgery, Department of Surgery, Cooper
University Hospital, Camden, New Jersey

ROBBIN G. COHEN, MD, MMM
Associate Professor of Cardiothoracic Surgery,
Department of Surgery, Keck School of
Medicine, University of Southern California,
Los Angeles, California

RAMSEY S. ELSAYED, MD
Research Assistant, Department of Surgery,
Keck School of Medicine, University of
Southern California, Los Angeles, California

ANTHONY ESTRERA, MD, FACS
Professor and Chief of Cardiac Surgery,
Department of Cardiothoracic and Vascular
Surgery, McGovern Medical School at The
University of Texas Health Science Center at
Houston (UTHealth) and Memorial Hermann
Hospital, Houston, Texas

FERNANDO FLEISCHMAN, MD
Assistant Professor, Associate Program
Director, Cardiothoracic Surgery, Co-Director,
Keck Aortic Center, Division of Cardiothoracic
Surgery, Department of Surgery,
CardioVascular Thoracic Institute, Keck School
of Medicine, University of Southern California,
Los Angeles, California

SUNG W. HAM, MD
Assistant Professor of Clinical Surgery, Division
of Vascular Surgery, Department of Surgery,
Keck School of Medicine, University of
Southern California, Los Angeles, California

SUKGU M. HAN, MD
Assistant Professor of Clinical Surgery, Division
of Vascular Surgery and Endovascular
Therapy, Department of Surgery, Keck School
of Medicine, University of Southern California,
Los Angeles, California

DAWN S. HUI, MD
Department of Surgery, Center for
Comprehensive Cardiovascular Care, Saint
Louis University, St Louis, Missouri

GEORGE JUSTISON, CCP
Manager, Perfusion Services, Perioperative
Services, University of Colorado Hospital,
Aurora, Colorado

ERIC C. KUO, MD
Research Resident, Division of Vascular
Surgery and Endovascular Therapy,
Department of Surgery, Keck School of
Medicine, University of Southern California,
Los Angeles, California

PAUL MICHAEL McFADDEN, MD
Professor of Clinical Cardiothoracic Surgery,
Surgical Co-Director of Lung Transplantation,
Division of Cardiothoracic Surgery, Keck
School of Medicine, University of Southern
California, Los Angeles, California

KAROL MEYERMANN, MD
Division of Vascular Surgery, Department of
Surgery, Cooper University Hospital, Camden,
New Jersey

MATTHEW S. MOSCA, CCP
Perfusionist, Perfusion Services, University of
Colorado Hospital, Aurora, Colorado

THOMAS BRETT REECE, MD
Associate Professor, Thoracic Aortic Surgery
Program, Division of Cardiothoracic Surgery,
Department of Surgery, University of Colorado
Anschutz Medical Campus, Aurora, Colorado

JACK C.J. SUN, MD, MS
Clinical Associate Professor of Surgery,
Division of Cardiothoracic Surgery, Keck
School of Medicine, University of Southern
California, Los Angeles, California

AKIKO TANAKA, MD, PhD
Department of Cardiothoracic and Vascular
Surgery, McGovern Medical School at The
University of Texas Health Science Center at
Houston (UTHealth) and Memorial Hermann
Hospital, Houston, Texas

PEDRO G.R. TEIXEIRA, MD
Associate Professor of Surgery, Department of
Surgery and Perioperative Care, Dell Medical
School, University of Texas at Austin, Austin,
Texas

MARC D. TRUST, MD
Chief Administrative Surgical Resident,
Department of Surgery and Perioperative Care,
Dell Medical School, University of Texas at
Austin, Austin, Texas

LUKE M. WIGGINS, MD
Division of Cardiothoracic Surgery,
Keck School of Medicine,
University of Southern California,
Los Angeles, California

GIORGIO ZANOTTI, MD
Division of Cardiothoracic Surgery,
Department of Surgery, University of
Colorado Anschutz Medical Campus, Aurora,
Colorado

Contents

Endovascular approaches to the aortic arch are challenged by unique anatomy and physiology of this area. Simple application of conventional endovascular technology and technique for abdominal or descending thoracic aortic disease to the aortic arch is insufficient to achieve effective and durable repairs. Appreciation of these challenges has led to developments in endovascular technology as well as complex strategies to deal with individual patient anatomy that hold the potential for continued improved outcomes in both the short and the long term.

Endovascular aortic repair to treat aortic arch abnormality has rapidly expanded in the last 2 decades, and surgeons now have options to treat patients who are poor candidates for open surgery. The devices and techniques should be tailored to the extension of the aortic abnormality and anatomy of the individual. Recent studies demonstrate promising results with branched endografts, but one of the major drawbacks of the devices is that considerable time is required to prepare the custommade graft, which may not be available for emergent or urgent cases. Introduction of commercially available devices is forthcoming.

Aortic arch surgery remains one of the most technically challenging procedures in cardiac surgery. It demands consideration of myocardial, brain, spinal cord, and lower body protection and rigorous surgical technique. Novel surgical approaches and refinements in brain and end organ protection strategies, liberal use of antegrade cerebral perfusion and moderate hypothermia have made arch repair safer. As endovascular technology and open surgical techniques evolve, aortic surgeons will need to continue to learn and incorporate these methods into practice in order to improve outcomes.

Stanford type B aortic dissections (TBADs) involve the descending aorta and can present with complications, including malperfusion syndrome or aortic rupture, which are associated with significant morbidity and mortality if left untreated. Clinical diagnosis is straightforward, typically confirmed using CT angiography. Treatment begins with immediate anti-impulse medical therapy. Acute TBAD with complications should be repaired with emergent thoracic endovascular aortic repair (TEVAR). Uncomplicated TBAD with high-risk features should undergo TEVAR in the subacute phase. Open surgical repair is seldom required and reserved only for select cases. It is critical to follow these patients clinically and radiographically in the outpatient setting.

Thoracoabdominal aortic aneurysms are increasing in incidence. Rupture is associated with a high rate of morbidity and mortality. The historic gold standard of open repair can be performed with low rates of complications at centers of excellence. However, these results are not universally achievable, with significantly higher rates of mortality reported from statewide studies. With the advent of endovascular therapy, techniques to mitigate the physiologic stress of open surgery have been developed. Hybrid open/endovascular operations are being undertaken with total visceral debranching followed by endografting. Totally endovascular procedures are now being performed using fenestrated, branched, and parallel endografts.

Treatment of Abdominal Aortic Pathology

Karol Meyermann and Francis J. Caputo

Abdominal aortic pathology is a diverse topic, ranging through a broad span of possible pathologies. The treatment options are equally vast, particularly with the ever-expanding endovascular techniques. In this article, we discuss management strategies for abdominal aortic aneurysms and aortic occlusive disease, because they represent some of the most common pathologies encountered in clinical scenarios.

Blunt Trauma of the Aorta, Current Guidelines

Marc D. Trust and Pedro G.R. Teixeira

Blunt thoracic aortic injury remains a major cause of prehospital deaths. For patients who reach the hospital alive, diagnosis and management have undergone dramatic changes over the last 50 years. Computed tomography scanning is the imaging modality of choice for injury diagnosis and repair planning. Medical management with antihypertensives dramatically decreases the risk of rupture, allowing for delayed repair, while abnormal physiology and more immediately life-threatening injuries can be addressed. Endovascular techniques and endograft technology have reduced significantly the risks associated with repair. However, the incidence of late complications associated with the devices currently available is not known.

Neuroprotection Strategies in Aortic Surgery

Edward J. Bergeron, Matthew S. Mosca, Muhammad Aftab, George Justison, and Thomas Brett Reece

Neurologic injury is a potentially devastating complication of aortic surgery. The methods used in aortic surgery, including systemic cooling, initiation of circulatory arrest, and rewarming during the replacement of the aortic arch, are the most complex circulatory management and surgical procedures performed in modern-day surgery. Despite the plethora of published literature, neuroprotection in aortic surgery is largely based on observational studies and institutional-based practices. This article summarizes the current evidence and emerging strategies for neuroprotection in aortic arch operations.

CARDIOLOGY CLINICS

Preface
Aortic Disease: Past and Present

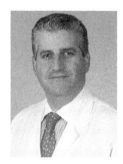

Fernando Fleischman, MD
Editor

Aortic diseases are a significant cause of morbidity and mortality in the Western world. The spectrum of aortic disease encompasses genetic disease syndromes as well as chronic disease control. It is expected that aortic diseases will continue to increase as the population ages. Education as to diagnosis and treatment is essential to treat these patients. Proper and prompt diagnosis is the cornerstone of aortic disease treatment. Malperfusion and rupture are uniquely morbid events that affect these patients when diagnosis is delayed.

It is a unique pleasure to introduce this issue of *Cardiology Clinics*. The issue covers the aorta from beginning to end. We deal with historical context as well as genetic causes. Articles focus on long-standing therapies and new endovascular techniques as well as future therapies. We begin with a thorough review of the history of aortic surgery. We then overview genetic disease states, followed by articles on each anatomic section of the aorta. From aortic root pathology to abdominal aortic disease states, the entirety of the aorta is covered by those who see these patients daily.

It is my hope that the articles in this issue cover the gamut of aortic disease. They elucidate the unique challenges facing the medical professional who treats these patients. I also believe that treating aortic disease crosses specialties in a way that furthers the need for multidisciplinary patient care. The team approach to care that brings radiologist, cardiac surgeons, cardiologists, and vascular surgeons to the table together improves patient outcomes. Collaboration is essential in the care of the aortic patient. On a personal note, I wish to express my immense gratitude to the editors and staff at *Cardiology Clinics*, who with their immense talent have brought this issue to life.

Fernando Fleischman, MD
Cardiothoracic Surgery
Keck Aortic Center
Division of Cardiothoracic Surgery
CardioVascular Thoracic Institute
Keck School of Medicine
University of Southern California
Los Angeles, CA 90033, USA

E-mail address:
fernando.fleischman@med.usc.edu

Cardiol Clin 35 (2017) xi
http://dx.doi.org/10.1016/j.ccl.2017.05.001
0733-8651/17/© 2017 Published by Elsevier Inc.

A History of Thoracic Aortic Surgery

Paul Michael McFadden, MD[a],*, Luke M. Wiggins, MD[a], Joshua A. Boys, MD[b]

KEYWORDS

• History • Aortic surgery • Thoracic aorta

KEY POINTS

- Ancient historical texts describe the presence of aortic pathologic conditions, although the surgical treatment of thoracic aortic disease remained insurmountable until the 19th century.
- Surgical treatment of thoracic aortic disease then progressed along with advances in surgical technique, conduit production, cardiopulmonary bypass, and endovascular technology.
- Despite radical advances in aortic surgery, principles established by surgical pioneers of the 19th century hold firm to this day.

There is no disease more conducive to clinical humility than aneurysm of the aorta.
—Sir William Osler

INTRODUCTION

A history of thoracic aortic surgery echoes the names of "giants" in medicine who through experience, anatomic and physiologic observation, laboratory and clinical experimentation, and sometimes even serendipitous discovery have independently and collectively contributed to our understanding of vascular surgery and ultimately to the surgical treatment of life-threatening aortic diseases. Progress in this area also depended on several advances made in other fields of medicine and surgery.

This article chronicles the important historical milestones in the development of current surgical and interventional management of thoracic aortic diseases as observed in the period of rapid progression in cardiac and thoracic surgery.[1,2]

EARLY HISTORY

Thoracic aortic surgery has its roots in the history of vascular surgery. Studies on Egyptian mummies found that arteriosclerosis and vascular calcification were relatively common 3500 years ago. However, most of our knowledge is derived from early historical accounts of treatment of vascular injuries in warfare and from management of peripheral extremity aneurysms. An early text, *Sushruta Samhita*, by Indian surgeon Sushruta (800–600 BC) provides one of the earliest descriptions of hemorrhage control by application of boiling oil, cautery, and the packing or ligation of vessels with hemp. Hindu surgeons of the day used "catgut" ligature to control bleeding vessels. The Greek physician Rufus (98–117 AD) described the control of vascular hemorrhage by digital compression, torsion of the artery, application of styptics, and arterial ligation. Galen, a Greek physician (second century AD) and surgeon to the early gladiators of Rome is said to have saved all of his gladiators by being the first to ligate their hemorrhaging arteries and applying styptics to venous bleeding. Antyllus, another celebrated Greek physician of that time, first described the course and treatment of peripheral arterial aneurysms. He described the difference between true and false aneurysms. He was first to describe the technique of proximal and distal ligation of aneurysms and evacuation of the aneurysm sac.[3,4]

a Division of Cardiothoracic Surgery, Keck School of Medicine, University of Southern California, 1520 San Pablo Street, Suite 4300, Los Angeles, CA 90033, USA; b Department of Surgery, Keck School of Medicine, University of Southern California, 1520 San Pablo Street, Suite 4300, Los Angeles, CA 90033, USA
* Corresponding author.
E-mail address: mmcfadden@surgery.usc.edu

Cardiol Clin 35 (2017) 307–316
http://dx.doi.org/10.1016/j.ccl.2017.03.001
0733-8651/17/© 2017 Elsevier Inc. All rights reserved.

VASCULAR AND AORTIC SURGERY RENAISSANCE

Advances in vascular and aneurysm surgery lay dormant for almost a millennium until Ambroise Pare' (1510–1590), a French military surgeon, reintroduced the concept of ligature of injured vessels and first described a ruptured thoracic aortic aneurysm. He alluded to the diagnostic and therapeutic challenges that thoracic aortic aneurysms posed to the surgical field in the coming centuries when he wrote, "The aneurysms that happen in the internal parts are incurable".[5–7] Pare's contemporary, Andreas Vesalius (1514–1564), a Flemish surgeon, was first to describe thoracic and abdominal aortic aneurysms.[8] Further advances in the description of the etiology and pathology of aortic aneurysms were published in 1728 by Lancisi in his text, *De Motu et Aneurysmatibus*.[9]

These early descriptions and grave prognostic outcomes posed a monumental challenge to surgical intervention for thoracic aortic aneurysms and aortic conditions in general. Several hundred years would pass before the earliest attempts at an operative intervention by British surgeon Moore in 1864. He described thrombosis of an ascending aneurysm of the thoracic aorta by the introduction of wire threads.[10] This thrombosis technique, marginal at best, persisted as the standard for operative management of aneurysms well in to the latter half of the 19th century. Attempts at improving the wiring process were carried out by Alfonso Corradi in 1879 who attached wires to a battery to induce coagulation of the aneurysm.[11] The results of this electrical-induced coagulation were imprecise and unimpressive until the early 20th century when Blakemore and King devised a precise method for electrothermic coagulation, which was published in *Journal of the American Medical Association* in 1938.[12] Another technique used by Harrison and Chandy in 1938 to indirectly treat thoracic aortic aneurysms included wrapping the aneurysm with cellophane to induce periarterial fibrosis and reinforce the aneurysm wall.[13] The results of this technique were inconsistent and it rapidly fell from favor.

ERA OF DISCOVERY AND INNOVATION

Alexis Carrel (**Fig. 1**), a celebrated French-born scientist and surgeon, began some of the earliest research and scientific investigations in organ transplantation and tissue culture in the late 1800s and early 1900s. He relocated from his home in Lyon, France to the United States hoping for a better opportunity to advance his work and was ultimately given a position at the Rockefeller

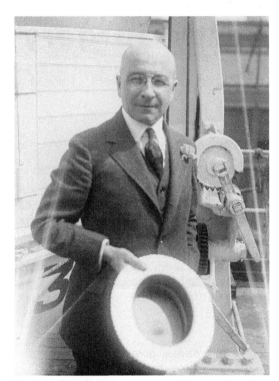

Fig. 1. Alexis Carrel. (*Courtesy of* George Grantham Bain Collection/Library of Congress, Washington, DC, Digital file no. ggbain 34418; with permission.)

Institute of Medical Research. Carrel is best known for his innovative and detailed work on suture technique for vascular anastomoses. His triangular or spatulated approach prevented the dreaded complications of stenosis, thrombosis, and leakage. This technique is still used by surgeons today. In a report Carrel presented to the American Surgical Association in 1910, he detailed his experimental work in this area. As a result, he was awarded the Nobel Prize in Physiology and Medicine in 1912. Another valuable contribution was his introduction of a chlorine-based topical antiseptic solution that he developed with his friend, English chemist H.D. Dakin. This solution was used extensively for wound care, in the absence of antibiotics, during World War I. In the 1930s he and famed aviator Charles Lindberg collaborated on the development of an early circulatory perfusion device to aid in organ preservation for transplantation.[3–8,14]

Rudolph Matas (1860–1957)

Rudolph Matas (**Fig. 2**) is considered a remarkable pioneer and leader in vascular surgery. He received his medical education and surgical training as a junior faculty member at the University of Louisiana, now Tulane University, in New

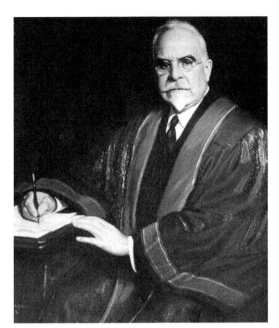

Fig. 2. Rudolph Matas in presidential robes. (*Courtesy of* the Archives of the American College of Surgeons, Chicago, IL; with permission.)

Orleans. Charity Hospital in New Orleans was considered a leading and highly respected medical community in the United States at the turn of the century. Matas, as a young faculty member was selected to travel to Cuba and investigate the Yellow Fever epidemic of the day and participated in identifying its transmission by a mosquito vector. In 1888, as an innovative young faculty surgeon, he introduced a successful operation to repair a traumatic brachial artery aneurysm on a man at Charity Hospital. Matas's famous operation entitled *Endoaneurysmorrhaphy* was reminiscent of an ancient procedure described by Antyllus, the second century Greek surgeon. It included proximal and distal ligation of the artery supplying the aneurysm, incision and resection of the sac and thrombus contents, and individual suture ligation of the feeding collateral vessels from within the sac. This surgery resulted in a marked reduction in extremity gangrene, as it preserved the external collateral blood flow to the distal extremity below the aneurysm. In 1895 at the age of 35, Matas was named Professor and Chairman of the Department of Surgery at Tulane. In 1923, Matas was the first to successfully ligate the aorta for an abdominal aortic aneurysm. He presided as the President of The American College of Surgeons from 1925 to 1926. As a result of these and other accomplishments, he is widely known as the Father of Vascular Surgery. Endoaneurysmorrhaphy was

abandoned by many with the introduction of synthetic tube grafts to replace the aneurysm, which became available in the 1950s. However, this technique was reintroduced by some surgeons for special indications, most notably Denton Cooley of Houston, Texas.[3,14–19]

IMPORTANT CONCURRENT DISCOVERIES

To arrive at the next evolution in the development of thoracic aortic surgery, several interdependent discoveries would be required. These occurred in the late 19th and mid-20th century, in part because of the advancements in the management of thromboembolism and developments in anticoagulation. In 1872, Trendelenburg, a celebrated German surgeon, recognized the high mortality rate associated with pulmonary embolism and devised a bedside technique to open the pulmonary artery and remove the embolism in postsurgical patients. The results of the Trendelenburg Procedure were not good.[3] However, in 1924 Martin Kirschner, a former pupil of Trendelenburg, performed and reported the first successful pulmonary embolectomy to the German Surgical Congress in Berlin. This report stirred much enthusiasm. A young visiting surgical resident from America, Alton Ochsner, was in attendance and was not impressed with the results reported. He felt the emphasis should be on prevention and not just a therapeutic reaction to remove thromboembolism.[20] In 1932, as surgery Professors at Tulane, Ochsner and Michael DeBakey advocated prophylactic inferior vena cava ligation instead. The same year, while a surgical resident and research fellow in Philadelphia, John Gibbon Jr. observed a heroic but unsuccessful attempt at a pulmonary embolectomy on a young woman. This traumatic and unfortunate case became the seminal event that resulted in Gibbon's development of the circulatory support device (**Fig. 3**). The Pump took Gibbon 21 years to develop, and in May 1953 he performed the first open heart surgery on extracorporeal support, a successful closure of an atrial septal defect in a young woman. A modification of the Trendelenburg operation using cardiopulmonary bypass support proved much more successful.[21]

Concurrent with the development of cardiopulmonary bypass, John McLean, an academic surgeon at Johns Hopkins Medical School, discovered heparin, which opened the door for therapeutic and prophylactic anticoagulation.[22] This discovery paved the way for extracorporeal perfusion thus ushering in the golden era of vascular, aortic, and open heart surgery.

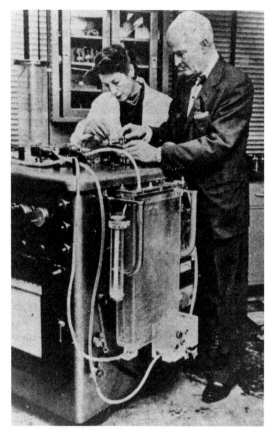

Fig. 3. John H. Gibbon, Mary H. Gibbon, and heart-lung machine. (*Courtesy of* Thomas Jefferson University, Archives and Special Collections, Philadelphia, PA; with permission.)

Alton Ochsner, MD (1896–1981)

In 1927, Alton Ochsner (**Fig. 4**) succeeded Rudolph Matas as Chairman of Surgery at Tulane University School of Medicine. Ochsner was an accomplished and internationally respected surgeon for his outstanding contributions in appendicitis, subphrenic abscess, and thrombophlebitis; however, he was best known for his pioneering work on lung cancer.[20–22] He was the first to identify cigarette smoking as a cause of lung cancer. He and his close surgical associate, Michael DeBakey, whom he mentored through medical school and surgical residency, were first to publish on this association and their surgical experience with lung cancer resections.[23–25] As a medical student, DeBakey developed the first roller pump, which was initially used for blood transfusion but later evolved into the roller pump used in cardiopulmonary bypass machines.[26] Matas and Ochsner each encouraged DeBakey to pursue a career in thoracic surgery and research.

Michael DeBakey, MD (1908–2008)

In 1948, DeBakey (see **Fig. 4**) left Tulane and moved to Houston, Texas to assume the position of Chairman of the Department of Surgery at the Baylor College of Medicine. This marked the passing of the torch of advances in thoracic aortic surgery to DeBakey and the incredible team he assembled and directed in Houston. In 1951, Denton Cooley joined the Baylor faculty and subsequently many other noted vascular and cardiac surgeons such as Crawford, Beal, Garrett, and Noon. During the early transition, the faculties of Baylor and Tulane collaborated and published on several important thoracic and vascular issues of the day.[27–40]

This collaboration among these institutions stemmed from a lifelong mentor relationship of Dr DeBakey with Alton Ochsner. DeBakey once shared an account of a particular experience in

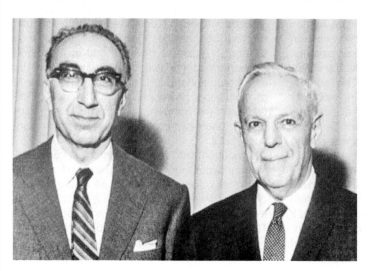

Fig. 4. Michael DeBakey (*left*) and Alton Ochsner (*right*). (*Photo courtesy of* Ochsner Medical Library and Archives, reproduced with permission, © OchsnerClinic Foundation.)

the operating room with Alton Ochsner that demonstrated his character as a leader and educator.

"A patient with an infected patent ductus arteriosus was being operated on in the Charity Hospital amphitheatre, which was filled with visiting surgeons attending a surgical congress in New Orleans. I was assisting Dr. Ochsner, and during the procedure and following his instructions, I was attempting to dissect and free up the aorta with my index finger on my side of the vessel in coordination with his effort on his side when I suddenly realized, with a gripping terror, that I had entered the aorta. The infection had made the wall of the vessel very friable. With a whisper that must have expressed my trepidation, I informed Dr. Ochsner of my concern. His equanimity and self-control were reflected in his calm response and his instruction to me to leave my finger there. He then deftly placed occluding sutures around the opening, and, as he tied the last suture, he asked me to remove my finger carefully. I am sure you can understand my sigh of relief in observing that there was no hemorrhage. He had met this challenge so skillfully that no one realized that a near fatal accident had occurred. Moreover, his understanding of my own dismay of this near fatal accident reflects his benevolence and magnanimous character, for after completion of the operation, he gave reassurances and commented kindly on my assistance."[24]

Denton A. Cooley, MD (1920–2016)

The celebrated American surgeon, Denton Cooley, was by all accounts a native Texan and a leader in cardiovascular surgery. Born in Houston, Texas, he graduated from the University of Texas where he also played college baseball and participated in fraternity life. He attended Johns Hopkins Medical School in Baltimore where he also did his surgical residency. His surgical training was temporarily interrupted for 2 years when called into service in the US Army Medical Corps during WW II, much like his colleague and mentor-to-be, Michael DeBakey. At Johns Hopkins, he assisted Alfred Blalock on the first Blue Baby operation, which stimulated his interest in congenital heart surgery. After studying a couple of years in London, Cooley returned to Houston to join DeBakey and the Baylor team. Immediately, the 2 surgeons began work on thoracic ascending, descending, arch aortic aneurysms, and brachiocephalic

vascular repairs.[41–45] Interestingly, John L. Ochsner, one of Alton Ochsner's 3 surgeon sons, trained under these 2 giants and became their lifelong friend and a highly respected cardiovascular surgeon and Chairman Emeritus of the Department of Surgery at the Ochsner Clinic in New Orleans. In 1952, Cooley was the first to perform the repair of a ruptured aortic aneurysm.[42] He and DeBakey then proceeded to perform firsts in almost all aspects of early thoracic aortic surgical repair.[46]

Norman E. Shumway, MD (1923–2006)

Norman Shumway (**Fig. 5**) was best known for his mentoring, research, and remarkably dedicated work in heart transplantation at Stanford University.[47,48] He performed the first human heart transplant in America and the second in the world in 1968, just 1 month after Christian Bernard's remarkable first transplant in Cape Town, South Africa. He received his undergraduate training at the University of Michigan and later at Baylor University in Waco, Texas. Shumway attended Vanderbilt University Medical School and received his Medical Degree in 1949. He completed surgical residency at the University of Minnesota under the famous C. Walt Lillehei and received a surgical doctorate in 1956. Shumway spent his entire academic career at Stanford University where he became Chairman of Stanford's Department of Cardiovascular and Thoracic Surgery. In addition to his seminal work on heart transplantation, Shumway was also a leader in the surgery of aortic dissection.[49–51] Shumway proposed a simple but more practical and widely embraced alternative classification to thoracic aortic dissections (**Fig. 6**; Stanford type A and type B).[52–54] It essentially replaced the more complex DeBakey classification. Shumway loved to operate, teach, and

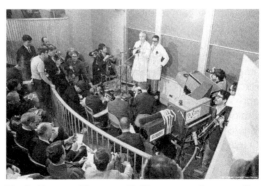

Fig. 5. Norman Shumway (left), press conference after first heart transplant. (*Courtesy of* Chuck Painter/ Stanford News Service.)

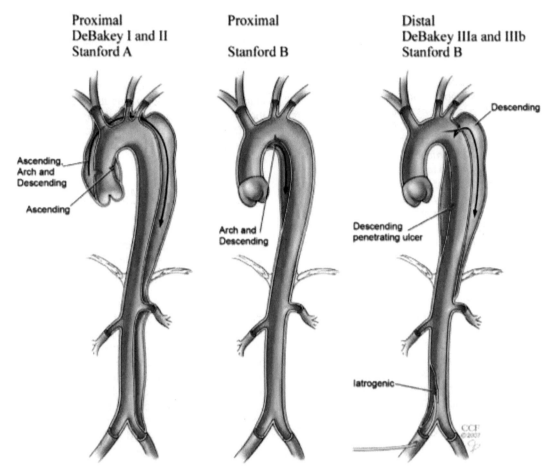

Fig. 6. Stanford and Debakey aortic classifications. (*Courtesy of* the Cleveland Clinic Foundation, Cleveland, OH; with permission.)

train his surgical residents and fellows. He surrounded himself with outstanding surgical faculty members, fellows, and residents. He promoted research and medical writing. Whenever a major surgical feat or advance was accomplished at Stanford, he would have the junior faculty or fellows involved take the credit and present the newsworthy item to the press. This act endeared him to those he trained, which included many surgeons who are noted for their work on surgical diseases of the aorta and who became leaders and surgical chairs at their respective universities: Randall Griepp (Mount Sinai), Larry Cohn (Brigham and Women's Hospital), Vaughn Starnes (USC), Craig Miller (Stanford) Bruce Reitz (Johns Hopkins/Stanford), and many more that have become giants in aortic surgery.

Hans Borst, MD

Hans Borst is a celebrated German surgeon and a leader in the development of surgery of aortic

arch dissections and repair of extensive thoracoabdominal aneurysms. Before the 1960s, operative intervention to the ascending aorta was well established. In 1963, Dr Borst was the first to successfully intervene on an arteriovenous fistula with an associated pseudoaneurysm of the aortic arch using circulatory arrest. Surgical intervention of the aortic arch became further established with the use of deep hypothermic circulatory arrest. Borst proceeded to invent a novel technique, the Elephant Trunk Procedure, for the management of aortic arch dissections and aneurysms that extended to the descending thoracic aorta. This procedure used a long aortic arch graft that was extended past the anastomosis of the distal aortic arch into the descending aorta for use in a subsequent staged operation for descending aortic replacement. This groundbreaking strategy was further modified to its modern equivalent, the Frozen Elephant Trunk Procedure, which is used most commonly today.[55–59]

Joseph Bavaria, MD

Dr Bavaria is a University of Pennsylvania–trained cardiothoracic surgeon and the Director of the institution's Aortic Center. He is also world renowned in the management of thoracic aortic disease and transcather aortic valve replacement and endovascular aortic interventional stenting. The discussion of Dr Bavaria's career leads us to the modern management of aortic pathologic conditions. He has played an integral role in the transition of open management of arch and descending thoracic aortic conditions to endovascular repair with stent grafting and hybrid procedures. His multiple articles show his vast experience in endovascular intervention and advocate the reduced morbidity and mortality often associated with endovascular technology.[60–65]

ADVANCES IN ENDOVASCULAR THERAPY

Dr Bavaria's work in the endovascular management of thoracic aortic conditions was preceded by a century of advances in radiographic and surgical technology. In 1903, Colt[66] pioneered the use of a small wire umbrella to be inserted through a cannula and expanded into an aneurysm. This approach, however, preceded most fundamentals of endovascular surgery. In 1924, the first arteriogram was performed by Barney Brookes. This arteriogram was performed to image the femoral artery, but the progression of endovascular surgery hinged on the ability to perform sophisticated imaging of the entire vascular tree.[67] The next 40 to 50 years ushered many advances in endovascular surgery, including the creation of the Fogarty embolectomy catheter, the first catheter-based arterial dilations, and the first vascular stent grafts.[68–70]

Parodi[71] was the first to conceive and construct a prototype of an aortic endovascular graft in the 1970s.[71] His ideas for an aortic graft gained popularity after he met and collaborated with Palmaz, who was a pioneer in the development of endovascular stents. Parodi was able to obtain the first US Food and Drug Administration approval for an endovascular stent design in the treatment of iliac arterial disease.[72] His first case with this device was performed in Argentina in 1990, which he later reported along with 4 additional cases in *Annals of Vascular Surgery* in 1991.[73]

Building on advances in the treatment of abdominal aneurysms, Dake and colleagues[74] reported the first thoracic endovascular aneurysm repair in 1994. Despite the lack of randomized controlled trials comparing open versus endovascular repair for thoracic aortic disease, endovascular repair was rapidly adopted because of significant improvement

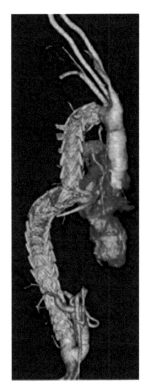

Fig. 7. Endovascular aortic repair. (*Reprinted with permission,* Cleveland Clinic Center for Medical Art & Photography © 2007–2017. All Rights Reserved.)

in early morbidity and mortality. Ultimately, the US Food and Drug Administration approved the first commercial device for thoracic endovascular aneurysm repair in 2005 (**Fig. 7**). Within the same decade, Dake and colleagues[74,75] published on the feasibility and efficacy of thoracic endovascular repair of both aneurysms and dissections. Bavaria and colleagues[60] demonstrated lower perioperative morbidity and mortality rates with comparable survival to standard open thoracic aortic aneurysm repair, which has lead to the emergence of preference for an endovascular approach.

SUMMARY

The late Harvard professor and Chief of Cardiac Surgery, Brigham Women's Hospital in Boston, Lawrence H. Cohn, MD, made an astute and reflective observation during the Annual American Association for Thoracic Surgery Meeting in 2010. He observed a phenomena, which was a welcome paradigm in every aspect of the thoracic and cardiovascular surgery academic program, technology conferences, plenary sessions, symposiums, papers, and exhibits, that there existed a strong collegial alliance and collaboration between the cardiothoracic surgeons, cardiologists, radiologists, vascular surgeons and biomedical engineers to work together for a common goal and to solve difficult issues facing the patients we serve. Through his and others' eyes, the traditional silos of independent specialties were being replaced by cooperative and collaborative service-line efforts, which better served all specialties and our patients.[76]

In a way, it is reminiscent of the cooperation, mentorship, and leadership that surgeons and others in related specialties observe in their own celebrated leaders. The giants in thoracic aortic surgery and endovascular intervention, whom we have just discussed, benefited enormously from the accomplishments of those who preceded them and the baton is now passed to the next generation of giants.

If I have seen further it is by standing on the shoulders of giants.
— Isaac Newton 1675

REFERENCES

1. Ochsner JL. Giants (presidential address). J Thorac Cardiovasc Surg 1993;106:769–78.
2. Ochsner A. The influence of serendipity on medicine. J Med Assoc State Ala 1946;15:347–66.
3. Westaby S. Surgery of the thoracic aorta. In: Westaby S, Bosher C, editors. Landmarks in cardiac surgery. Oxford (England): Isis Medical Media; 1997. p. 223–52.
4. Thompson JE. Early history of aortic surgery. J Vasc Surg 1998;28:746–52.
5. Barker WF. Clio: the arteries. Austin (TX): RG Landers; 1992. p. 2–502.
6. Paget S. Ambroise Pare and his times, 1510-1590. New York: G.P. Putnam's Sons; 1897. p. 26. Accessed November 2, 2012.
7. Paré A. A surgeon in the field. In: Ross JB, McLauglin MM, editors. The portable renaissance reader. New York: Viking Penguin; 1981. p. 558–63.
8. Slaney G. A history of aneurysm surgery. In: Greenhalgh RM, Mannick JA, Powell JT, editors. The cause and management of aneurysms. London: WB Saunders; 1990. p. 1–18.
9. Wright WC, editor. Lancisi GM: De Aneurysmatibus. New York: Macmillan; 1952.
10. Moore CH, Murchison C. On a method procuring the consolidation of fibrin in certain incurable aneurysms: with a report of a case in which an aneurysm of the ascending aorta was treated by the insertion of wire. (London 1864). Med ChirTrans 1864;47:129–49.
11. Osler W. The principles and practice of medicine. 7th edition. New York: D. Appleton; 1909. p. 862–3.
12. Blakemore A, King BG. Electrothermic coagulation of aortic aneurysms. JAMA 1938;111:1821–7.
13. Harrison PW, Chandy J. A subclavian aneurysm cured by a cellophane fibrosis. Ann Surg 1943;118:478–81.
14. Akerman J. Nobel lectures; physiology or medicine 1901-1921. Amsterdam: Elsevier Publishing Company; 1967.
15. Haimovici H. A historical overview of vascular surgery: past record and new trends- Avision for the 1990's. In: Haimovici H, Ascer E, Hollier LH, et al, editors. Haimovici's vascular surgery. Cambridge (MA): Blackwell Science Inc; 1996. p. 1–2.
16. Livesay JJ, Messner GN, Vaughn WK. Milestones in the treatment of aortic aneusyms. Tex Heart Inst J 2005;32:130–4.
17. Ochsner J. The complex life of Rudolph Matas. J Vasc Surg 2001;34:387–92.
18. Matas R. Traumatic aneurysm of the left brachial artery. Incision and partial incision of the sac- recovery. Med News New York 1888;53:462–6.
19. Matas R. An operation for the radical cure of aneurysm based upon arteriorrhaphy. Ann Surg 1903;37:161–96.
20. McFadden PM, Ochsner JL. A history of the diagnosis and treatment of venous thrombosis and pulmonary embolism. Ochsner J 2002;4:9–13.
21. Sharp EH. Pulmonary embolectomy: successful removal of a massive pulmonary embolus with the support of cardiopulmonary bypass. Case Report. Ann Surg 1962;156:1–4.
22. McLean J. The discovery of heparin. Circulation 1959;19:75–8.
23. Porter GH. Alton Ochsner. The man and his contributions. Med Clin North Am 1992;76:1007–13.
24. Ventura HO. Alton Ochsner, MD: physician. Ochsner J 2002;4:48–52.
25. Wilds J, Harkey I. Alton ochsner surgeon of the south. Baton Rouge (LA): Louisiana State University Press; 1990.
26. DeBakey ME. A continous flow blood transfusion instrument. New Orleans Med Surg J 1934;87:386–9.
27. Ochsner A, DeBakey M. Primary pulmonary malignancy: treatment by total pneumonectomy; analysis of 79 collected cases and 7 personal cases. Surg Gynecol Obstet 1939;48:433–51.
28. Ochsner A, DeBakey M. Carcinoma of the lung. Arch Surg 1941;42:209–58.
29. Ochsner A, DeBakey M, Dixon L. Primary pulmonary malignancy treated by resection: an analysis of 129 cases. Ann Surg 1947;125(5):522.
30. DeBakey ME, Cooley DA, Creech O Jr. Surgical treatment of aneurysms and occlusive disease of the aorta. Postgrad Med 1954;15:120–7.
31. DeBakey ME, Creech O. Surgical treatment of epiphrenic diverticulum of the esophagus. J Thorac Surg 1952;23:486–94.
32. Ochsner A, DeCamp PT, DeBakey ME, et al. Bronchogenic carcinoma: its frequency, diagnosis

and early treatment. J Am Med Assoc 1952;148: 691–7.

33. Ochsner A, DeBakey ME, DeCamp PT, et al. Broncogenic carcinoma. Med Arts Sci 1952;6:1–8.

34. DeCamp PT, Laundry RM, Ochsner A, et al. Spontaneous thrombophlebitis. Surgery 1952;31:43–54.

35. Ochsner A, DeBakey ME, DeCamp PT, et al. Thromboembolism: an analysis of cases at the Charity hospital in new Orleans over a 12-year period. Ann Surg 1951;134:405–19.

36. Ochsner A, De Camp PT, DeBakey ME. Venous thrombosis. Ann West Med Surg 1951;5:705–8.

37. DeBakey ME, Ochsner A. Hepatic amebiasis: a 20 year experience and analysis of 263 cases. Surg Gynecol Obste 1951;92:209–31.

38. Orime Y, Takatani S, Shiono M, et al. Versatile one-piece total artificial heart for bridge to transplantation or permanent heart replacement. Artif Organs 1992;16:607–12.

39. Tayama E, Olsen DB, Ohashi Y, et al. The DeBakey ventricular assist device: current status in 1997. Artif Organs 1999;23:1113–6.

40. Mcfadden PM, Ochsner JL. Surgical technique for aortic dissection. In: Jamieson CW, Yao JST, editors. Rob and smiths operative surgery, vascular surgery. 5th edition. London: Chapman & Hall; 1994. p. 163–79.

41. Cooley DA, De Bakey ME. Surgical considerations of intrathoracic aneurysms of the aorta and great vessels. Ann Surg 1952;135:660–80.

42. Cooley DA, DeBakey ME. Ruptured aneurysms of abdominal aorta; excision and homograft replacement. Postgrad Med 1954;16:334–42.

43. Cooley DA, DeBakey ME. Successful resection of aneursym of thoracic aorta and replacement by graft. JAMA 1953;152:673–6.

44. Cooley DA, DeBakey ME. Resection of entire ascending aorta in fusiform aneurysm using cardiac bypass. JAMA 1956;162:1158–9.

45. DeBakey ME, Crawford ES, Cooley DA, et al. Successful resection of fusiform aneurysm of aortic arch with replacement by homograft. Surg Gynecol Obstet 1957;105:657–64.

46. Cooley DA. A brief history of aortic aneurysm surgery. Aorta (Stamford) 2013;1:1–3.

47. Griepp RB, Stinson EB, Shumway NE. Transplantation of the heart. Surg Annu 1976;8:47–62, 1974.

48. Shumway NE, Dong E Jr, Stinson EB, et al. The Stanford University experience with clinical heart transplantation (author's transl). Nihon Kyobu Geka Gakkai Zasshi 1974;22:787–95.

49. Fann JI, Smith JA, Miller DC, et al. Surgical management of aortic dissection during a 30-year period. Circulation 1995;92:113–21.

50. Smith JA, Fann JI, Miller DC, et al. Surgical management of aortic dissection in patients with the Marfan syndrome. Circulation 1994;90:235–42.

51. Yun KL, Glower DD, Miller DC, et al. Aortic dissection resulting from tear of transverse arch: is concomitant arch repair warranted? J Thorac Cardiovasc Surg 1991;102:355–68.

52. Lai DT, Miller DC, Mitchell RS, et al. Acute type A aortic dissection complicated by aortic regurgitation: composite valve graft versus separate valve graft versus conservative valve repair. J Thorac Cardiovasc Surg 2003;126:1978–86.

53. Umana JP, Lai DT, Mitchell RS, et al. Is medical therapy still the optimal treatment strategy for patients with acute type B aortic dissection? J Thorac Cardiovasc Surg 2002;124:896–910.

54. Lai DT, Robbins RC, Mitchell RS, et al. Does profound hypothermic circulatory arrest improve survival in patients with acute type A aortic dissection? Circulation 2002;106:218–28.

55. Borst HG, Shaudig A, Rudolph W. Arteriovenous fistula of the aortic arch repair during deep hypothermia and circulatory arrest. J Thorac Cardiovasc Surg 1964;48:443–7.

56. Borst HG, Walterbusch G, Schaps D. Extensive aortic replacement using "elephant trunk" prosthesis. J Thorac Cardiovasc Surg 1983;31:37–40.

57. Crawford ES, Saleh SA, Schwessler JS. Treatment of aneurysms of the transverse aortic arch. J Thorac Cardiovasc Surg 1979;78:383–93.

58. Svensson LG. Rationale and technique for replacement of the ascending aorta, arch, and distal aorta using a modified elephant trunk procedure. J Card Surg 1992;7:301–12.

59. Karck M, Charvan A, Khaladj N, et al. The frozen elephant trunk technique for the treatment of extensive thoracic aneurysms: operative results and follow up. Eur J Cardiothorac Surg 2005;28:286–90.

60. Bavaria JE, Appoo JJ, Makaroun MS, et al, Gore TAG Investigators. Endovascular stent grafting versus open surgical repair of descending thoracic aortic aneurysms in low-risk patients: a multicenter comparative trial. J Thorac Cardiovasc Surg 2007; 133(2):369–77.

61. Kouchoukos NT, Bavaria JE, Coselli JS, et al. Guidelines for credentialing of practitioners to perform endovascular stent-grafting of the thoracic aorta. J Thorac Cardiovasc Surg 2006;131(3):530–2.

62. Appoo JJ, Moser WM, Fairman RM, et al. Thoracic aortic stent grafting: improving results with newer generation investigational devices. J Thorac Cardiovasc Surg 2006;131(5):1087–94.

63. Szeto WY, Bavaria JE, Bowen FW, et al. The hybrid total arch repair: brachiocephalic bypass and concomitant endovascular aortic arch stent graft placement. J Card Surg 2007;22(2):97–102.

64. Szeto WY, Bavaria JE, Bowen FW, et al. Reoperative aortic root replacement in patients with previous aortic surgery. Ann Thorac Surg 2007;84(5):1592–8 [discussion: 1598–9].

65. Szeto WY, Bavaria JE. Advances in thoracic endo-vascular aortic repair: introduction. Semin Thorac Cardiovasc Surg 2009;21(4):339–40.

66. Colt GH. The clinical duration of saccular aortic aneurysm in British-born subjects. Q J Med 1927; 20:331–48.

67. Brooks B. Intra-arterial injection of sodium iodide: preliminary report. JAMA 1924;82:1016–9.

68. Fogarty TJ, Cranley JJ, Krause RJ, et al. A method for extraction of arterial emboli and thrombi. Surg Gynecol Obstet 1963;116:241–4.

69. Dotter CT, Judkins MP. Transluminal treatment of arteriosclerotic obstruction. Description of a new technic and preliminary report of its application. Circulation 1964;30:54–70.

70. Dotter CT. Transluminally-placed coilspring endarterial tube grafts. Long-term patency in canine popliteal artery. Invest Radiol 1969;4:329–32.

71. Parodi JC. Ten years of endovascular aneurysm repair. Endovascular Today 2007. Supplement, 4–5.

72. Palmaz J. The advent of stenting. Endovascular Today 2004;45–9.

73. Parodi JC, Palmaz JC, Barone HD. Transfemoral intraluminal graft implantation for abdominal aortic aneurysms. Ann Vasc Surg 1991;5:491–9.

74. Dake MD, Miller DC, Semba CP, et al. Transluminal placement of endovascular stent–grafts for the treatment of descending thoracic aortic aneurysms. N Engl J Med 1994;331:1729–34.

75. Dake MD, Kato N, Mitchell RS, et al. Endovascular stent-graft placement for the treatment of acute aortic dissection. Engl J Med 1999;340(20): 1546–52.

76. Cohn LH. The times they are a-changin'. J Thorac Cardiovasc Surg 2010;140:3–4.

Genetic Disorders of the Thoracic Aorta and Indications for Surgery

 CrossMark

Jack C.J. Sun, MD, MS*

KEYWORDS

- Aortic aneurysm • Genetic disorders • Connective tissue disease • Aortic surgery
- Marfan syndrome

KEY POINTS

- Genetic disorders of the aorta are rare but can be life threatening.
- Genetic causes of many connective tissue diseases are well defined.
- Familial thoracic aortic aneurysm and bicuspid aortic valve aortopathy are heritable, but their genetic causes are not well known.
- Natural history of genetic thoracic aortic aneurysms is not well understood or predictable, and surgical guidelines for treatment remain imprecise.

INTRODUCTION

Thoracic aortic aneurysm (TAA) can be a life-threatening condition affecting a broad range of patients from the young to the elderly. It is estimated that greater than 20% of all TAAs have a genetic basis.[1,2] These aneurysms are much more likely to affect the aortic root and ascending aorta as opposed to the atherosclerotic or degenerative TAAs where the descending thoracic aorta is more commonly involved. TAAs associated with an underlying genetic predisposition can be challenging to diagnose and treat. Genetic and molecular pathways contributing to the pathophysiology of these aneurysms are still not fully understood and continue to be studied, but much progress has been made. To determine when surgical repair is indicated, we must be familiar with the mechanisms and natural history of genetic disorders of the thoracic aorta.

MARFAN SYNDROME

Marfan syndrome (MFS) is an autosomal dominant connective tissue disorder caused by mutations in the fibrillin-1 (FBN1) gene. FBN1 is an extracellular matrix protein that plays a significant role in the strength and integrity of aortic tissue by promoting smooth muscle cell anchorage to elastin and collagen matrices.[3] FBN1 gene mutation leads to FBN1 deficiency and increased transforming growth factor-β (TGFB) leading to aortic inflammation and fibrosis and, ultimately, dilatation and aneurysm formation.[4] The ascending aorta, aortic root, and aortic annulus are the most commonly affected,[5] although the entire thoracic aorta can become aneurysmal over the lifetime of a patient with MFS. Clinically, MFS is diagnosed using the Ghent criteria.[6] A second locus for MFS (MFS2) is caused by mutations in TGFB receptor 2 (TGFBR2), forming a phenotype that likely shares characteristics with Loeys-Dietz syndrome (LDS).[7]

LOEYS-DIETZ SYNDROME

LDS is also an autosomal dominant connective tissue disorder caused by mutations in TGFBR1 and TGFBR2.[8] The severe weakening of the aortic tissue in LDS patients can lead to premature and

Disclosure Statement: The author has nothing to disclose.
Division of Cardiothoracic Surgery, University of Southern California, Keck School of Medicine, 1975 Zonal Avenue, Los Angeles, CA 90033, USA
* 2841 Lomita Boulevard, Suite 310, Torrance, CA 90505.
E-mail address: jack.sun@med.usc.edu

Cardiol Clin 35 (2017) 317–320
http://dx.doi.org/10.1016/j.ccl.2017.03.003
0733-8651/17/© 2017 Elsevier Inc. All rights reserved.

cardiology.theclinics.com

aggressive aneurysms. Aortic dissection can often occur in young patients and without significant aortic dilatation similar to what is seen in patients with Ehlers-Danlos syndrome (EDS). Patients with MFS aortic dissection, however, often have concomitant ascending and aortic root aneurysms.[9]

Phenotypically, patients with LDS exhibit thin translucent skin with visible veins, dystrophic scars, craniofacial deformities such as bifid uvula and hypertelorism, and easy bruising and joint laxity.[10]

EHLERS-DANLOS SYNDROME TYPE IV (VASCULAR TYPE)

EDS is an autosomal dominant connective tissue disorder caused by mutations in the type III procollagen (COL3A1) gene. This mutation leads to defective type III procollagen, the most amply represented type of collagen normally found in the extracellular matrix of the aorta.[11] Patients with vascular type EDS can have rupture of not just the aorta but also of smaller arteries. As previously mentioned, EDS patients, similar to LDS patients, can subsequently have aortic dissection with normal-sized aortas. Phenotypically, patients with EDS have thin skin with visible veins, easy bruising, thin pinched nose, thin lips, prominent ears, hollow cheeks, and tight facial skin.[11]

FAMILIAL THORACIC AORTIC ANEURYSM

A significant family history of TAAs puts a patient at significant increased risk for the condition. This is still a growing area of research and is more difficult clinically to ascertain, as patients do not have an associated syndrome of visible or examinable features. Up to 20% of TAAs are familial in origin, and there have been genetic factors discovered that are heterogeneous and with variable pentrance.[1] Genes found to be associated with familial TAAs include those responsible for the contractile apparatus of smooth muscle cells (ACTA2, MYH11, MYLK, PRKG1) and additional TGFB pathway proteins such as SMAD3.[12]

BICUSPID AORTIC VALVE AORTOPATHY

Approximately 1% to 2% of the population is born with a bicuspid aortic valve (BAV) in a 2:1 male/female ratio, thus representing the most common congenital heart defect.[5] The bicuspid aortic valve can present with phenotypically heterogeneous malformations with different fusion patterns.[13] Patients with BAV are less predictable in terms of the development or progression of TAA. They can have varying degrees of aortopathy, and this may

have a relationship with the BAV leaflet configuration. Those with a true bicuspid aortic valve with only 2 commissures and no raphe are less prone to aortic dilatation than those with fused leaflets and the presence of a raphe.[14]

BAV is usually not associated with genetic syndromes but can be found concomitantly with connective tissue disorders such as MFS, LDS, and EDS. BAV does run in families and is thus believed to be highly heritable, with 9% of first-degree relatives of people with BAV found to have the same congenital condition.[15] Despite this finding, a specific genetic defect has not been identified as a cause for BAV aortopathy. The inheritance pattern seems to be autosomal dominant with decreased penetrance and variable expressivity but may also have an X-linked etiology, as BAV occurs much more frequently in males. Multiple gene mutations are found to have an association in some BAV patients, but these familiar mutations may also represent an overlapping with thoracic familial thoracic aortic aneurysms or other genetic disorders. These gene mutations include NOTCH1, ACTA2, TFGB2, FBN1, KCNJ2, GATA5, Nkx2-5, and SMAD6.[16]

Patients with BAV aortopathy have a 25% to 35% risk of needing aortic surgery over their lifetime and a 53% risk of needing valve surgery.[13,17] Anatomically, approximately 50% of BAV patients who subsequently have TAA have enlargement of the aortic root and ascending aorta, 25% of the ascending aorta and arch, and 25% of either isolated aortic root or isolated ascending aorta.[18]

NATURAL HISTORY OF GENETIC CAUSES OF THORACIC AORTIC ANEURYSM

There are limited data documenting the natural history of patients with genetic disorders and TAAs because of their low incidence and limitations to study follow-up. Patients with MFS have a rate of growth of their TAAs of 0.5 to 1 mm per year. Familial TAAs can grow rapidly at 2.1 mm per year, whereas LDS can have rapid growth of greater than 10 mm per year. The rate of growth of the descending aorta is generally greater than that of the ascending aorta.[19] Patients with genetic disorders and familial TAAs have faster rates of growth of their aneurysms but also much higher incidences of rupture and dissection at smaller sizes.

Patients with BAV aortopathy can have rates of growth of their TAAs of 0.5 to 2 mm per year.[20] Although these TAAs grow faster than degenerative/hypertensive aneurysms, they have rates of rupture and dissection that are similar for their respective sizes.[17]

Table 1
Genetic disorders of the aorta

Genetic Disorder	Genetic Defect	Clinical Features	Size Indication for Surgery[a]
MS	FBN1 TGFBR2	Ghent criteria Skeletal features Ectopia lentis Dural ectasia	≥5.0 cm ≥4.5 cm with risk factors[b]
LDS	TGFBR1, TGFBR2	Translucent skin, dystrophic scars, bifid uvula, hypertelorism, easy bruising, join laxity	≥4.4 cm
EDS type IV (vascular type)	COL3A1	Translucent skin, easy bruising, thin pinched nose, prominent ears, hollow cheeks, tight facial skin	≥4.4 cm
Familial TAA	Some association with ACTA2, MYH11, PRKG1, SMAD3	None	No specific recommendation
BAV aortopathy	Some association with NOTCH1, ACTA2, TFGB2, FBN1, KCNJ2, GATA5, Nkx2-5, SMAD6	None but may be associated with genetic syndromes or other congenital heart disease	≥5.5 cm ≥5.0 cm with risk factors[c] ≥4.5 cm concomitant surgery

[a] Rate of growth ≥0.5 cm/y and symptomatic aortic aneurysm are indications for surgery for all types.
[b] Family history of aortic dissection, aortic size growth >3 mm/y, severe aortic or mitral regurgitation, desire for pregnancy.
[c] Coarctation of aorta, hypertension, family history of aortic dissection, aortic growth >3 mm/y.

INDICATIONS FOR SURGERY

Current indications for surgery are provided by guidelines put out by the American College of Cardiology/American Heart Association[20,21] and the European Society of Cardiology[19] (**Table 1**). There is unfortunately a paucity of data to provide a strong rationale for size cutoffs when it comes to determining the threshold to undergo surgery. Recommendations are mostly based on expert consensus and small case series. For patients with MFS, guidelines recommend surgery once the aortic diameter reaches 5.0 cm or 4.5 cm if additional risk factors exist (family history of aortic dissection, aortic size growth >3 mm/y, severe aortic or mitral regurgitation, or desire for pregnancy). For LDS and EDS, the European Society of Cardiology does not provide recommendations because of their perceived lack of available evidence, whereas the American College of Cardiology/American Heart Association recommends surgical repair once the aortic diameter reaches 4.4 cm.

Patients with BAV aortopathy are recommended for surgical repair once their aortic diameter reaches 5.5 cm or 5.0 cm in the presence of other risk factors (coarctation of aorta, hypertension, family history of aortic dissection, aortic growth >3 mm/y). At the time of concomitant cardiac surgery, an ascending or root aortic aneurysm size of 4.5 cm or greater should be strongly considered for repair.

SUMMARY

Genetic disorders of the aorta, although rare, can be devastating and substantially shorten the lifespan of those affected. Early diagnosis, close surveillance, and appropriate medical and surgical management are the keys to contemporary management, although improving outcomes and long-term survival in these patients proves challenging. Surgical guidelines based on aortic diameter sizes are likely oversimplified, as there are a substantial proportion of these patients who suffer fatal ruptures or dissection at sizes well less than these recommended cutoffs. Ongoing genetic research will help shed additional light on the underlying causes and mechanisms of these disorders. Future goals will include the ability to create genetic profiles that will allow us to determine a patient's individualized risk for an acute aortic event and thus provide customized treatment plans.

REFERENCES

1. Coady MA, Davies RR, Roberts M, et al. Familial patterns of thoracic aortic aneurysms. Arch Surg 1999; 134(4):361–7.
2. Albornoz G, Coady MA, Roberts M, et al. Familial thoracic aortic aneurysms and dissections-incidence, modes of inheritance, and phenotypic patterns. Ann Thorac Surg 2006;82(4):1400–5.
3. Dietz HC, Cutting GR, Pyeritz RE, et al. Marfan syndrome caused by a recurrent de novo missense mutation in the fibrillin gene. Nature 1991;352(6333):337–9.
4. Neptune ER, Frischmeyer PA, Arking DE, et al. Dysregulation of TGF-B activation tonributes to pathogenesis in Marfan syndrome. Nat Genet 2003; 33(3):407–11.
5. Paterick TE, Humphries JA, Ammar KA, et al. Aortopathies: etiologies, genetics, differential diagnosis, prognosis and management. Am J Med 2013;126:670–8.
6. Loeys BL, Dietz HC, Braverman AC, et al. The revised ghent nosology for the Marfan syndrome. J Med Genet 2010;47(7):476–85.
7. Collod G, Babron MC, Jondea G, et al. A second locus for Marfan syndrome maps to chromosome 3p24.2-p25. Nat Genet 1994;8(3):264–8.
8. Loeys BL, Schwarze U, Holm T, et al. Aneurysm syndromes caused by mutations in the TGF-B receptor. N Engl J Med 2006;355(8):788–98.
9. Iskandar A, Thompson PD. Diseases of the aorta in elite athletes. Clin Sports Med 2015;34:461–72.
10. Ikeda Y. Aortic aneurysm: etiopathogenesis and clinicopathologic correlations. Ann Vasc Dis 2016; 9(2):73–9.
11. Pepin M, Schwarze U, Superti-Furga A, et al. Clinical and genetic features of Ehlers-Danlos syndrome type IV, the vascular type. N Engl J Med 2000; 342(10):673–80.
12. Jondeau G, Boileau C. Familial thoracic aortic aneurysms. Curr Opin Cardiol 2014;29(6):492–8.
13. Freeze SL, Landis BJ, Ware SM, et al. Bicuspid aortic valve: a review with recommendations for genetic counseling. J Genet Couns 2016;25(6): 1171–8.
14. Kari FA, Beyersdorf F, Siepe M. Pathophysiological implications of different bicuspid aortic valve configurations. Cardiol Res Pract 2012;2012:735829.
15. Cripe L, Andelfinger G, Martin LJ, et al. Bicuspid aortic valve is heritable. J Am Coll Cardiol 2004;44: 138–43.
16. Andreassi MG, Della Corte A. Genetics of bicuspid aortic valve aortopathy. Curr Opin Cardiol 2016;31: 585–92.
17. Michelena HI, Khanna AD, Mahoney D, et al. Incidence of aortic complications in patients with bicuspid aortic valves. JAMA 2011;306:1104–12.
18. Fazel SS, Mallidi HR, Lee RS, et al. The aortopathy of bicuspid aortic valve disease has distinctive patterns and usually involves the transverse aortic arch. J Thorac Cardiovasc Surg 2008;135:901–7.
19. Erbel R, Aboyans V, Boileau C, et al. 2014 ESC Guidelines on the diagnosis and greatment of aortic diseases. Eur Heart J 2014;35:2873–926.
20. Nishimura RA, Otto CM, Bonow RO, et al. 2014 AHA/ACC Guidelines for the management of patients with valvular heart disease: a report of the American College of Cardiology/American Heart Association task force on practice guidelines. Circulation 2014; 129(23):e521–643.
21. Hirtazka LF, Bakris GL, Beckman JA, et al. 2010 ACCF/AHA/AATS/ACR/ASA/SCA/SCAI/SIR/STS/SVM Guidelines for the diagnosis and management of patients with thoracic aortic disease. Circulation 2010;121:e266–369.

Surgery for Diseases of the Aortic Root

Robbin G. Cohen, MD, MMM*, Ramsey S. Elsayed, MD, Michael E. Bowdish, MD

KEYWORDS

- Cardiac surgery • Aortic root • Diagnosis • Management • Outcomes

KEY POINTS

- The aortic root represents the outflow tract from the left ventricle where it acts as a bridge between the left ventricle and the ascending aorta.
- The aortic root comprises the aortic valve and the coronary ostia.
- Aortic root surgery is indicated in the setting of aneurysmal dilatation, acute aortic dissection, and acute endocarditis.
- Repair frequently involves the replacement of the aortic root including the aortic valve, which can include a prosthetic valve, cryopreserved homograft, or a pulmonary autograft.
- Many patients are candidates for aortic root reconstruction with valve sparing of the native aortic valve.

INTRODUCTION AND ANATOMY

The aortic root is the origin of the aorta, commencing where the ventricular musculature of the left ventricular outflow tract changes to that of the fibroblastic wall of the ventricular arterial junction.[1] It begins with the aortic annulus, the hemodynamic boundary between the left ventricle and the aorta, and ends at the sinotubular junction just distal to the aortic valve commissures (**Fig. 1**). It contains the aortic annulus, the aortic cusps, the aortic sinuses from which the coronary arteries originate, and the sinotubular junction, all of which function physiologically as a unit. The aortic annulus has a scalloped shape and is attached directly to myocardium in approximately 45% of its circumference and 55% to fibrous structures. The diameter of the aortic annulus is 10% to 20% larger than the diameter of the sinotubular junction in younger patients but becomes equal with age as its elastic fibers allow dilatation over time.

Leonardo da Vinci described the anatomy of the aortic root in 1513, depicting both the opened and closed aortic valve within the cylinder of the aorta.[2] In 1740, Valsalva correctly suggested that coronary artery filling takes place during diastole from these sinuses.[3] Since then, a fundamental understanding of the anatomic and functional relationships of the components of the aortic root have developed. These, in turn, have allowed for the development of sophisticated surgical procedures to both replace and reconstruct the aortic root, depending on the pathologic process. Tirone David, one of the world's authorities on the pathophysiology and surgical reconstruction of the aortic root, nicely described the relationships of the aortic valve cusps to each other and to the sinotubular junction: "During diastole, the free margins and part of the body of the three cusps touch each other approximately in the center of the aortic root to seal the aortic orifice. Thus the average length of the free margins of three aortic

Disclosure Statement: No authors have a relationship with a commercial entity with a direct financial interest in the subject matter or materials discussed in this article.
Department of Surgery, Keck School of Medicine of USC, University of Southern California, 1520 San Pablo Street, HCC II, Suite 4300, Los Angeles, CA 90033, USA
* Corresponding author.
E-mail address: Robbin.Cohen@med.usc.edu

cardiology.theclinics.com

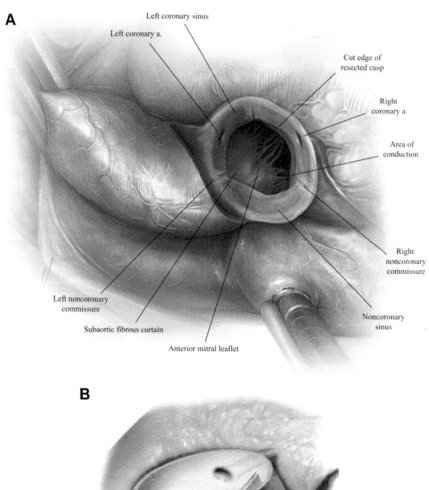

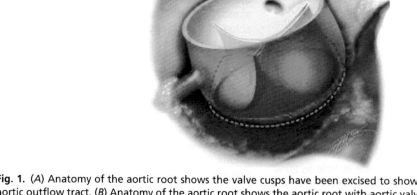

Fig. 1. (*A*) Anatomy of the aortic root shows the valve cusps have been excised to show the aortic annulus and aortic outflow tract. (*B*) Anatomy of the aortic root shows the aortic root with aortic valve intact. (*Adapted from* [*A*] Grubb, KJ. Aortic root enlargement during aortic valve replacement: nicks and manouguian techniques. Oper Tech Thorac Cardiovasc Surg 2015;20(3):206–18, with permission; and [*B*] Holubec T, Higashigaito K, Belobradek Z, et al. An expansible aortic ring in aortic root remodeling: exact position, pulsatility, effectiveness, and stability in three-dimensional CT study. Ann Thorac Surg 2017;103(1):83–90, with permission.)

cusps must exceed the diameter of the sinotubular junction to allow the cusps to coapt centrally and render the aortic valve competent. If a pathologic process causes shortening of the length of the free margin of a cusp or if the sinotubular junction dilates, the cusps cannot coapt centrally resulting in aortic insufficiency. If the length of a free margin is elongated, the cusp prolapses, and depending of the degree of prolapse, aortic insufficiency ensues."[4] Dilatation of the aortic root with and without aortic insufficiency is most commonly caused by abnormalities of the connective tissue of the aortic wall. These are frequently found in the genetically related connective tissue disorders, such as Marfan disease and the valvular and aortic wall abnormalities associated with bicuspid aortic valve. This article discusses the important diseases of the aortic root, and describes their surgical therapy.

INDICATIONS FOR AORTIC ROOT SURGERY

The most common indications for aortic root surgery are aneurysmal dilatation with or without aortic valve disease, acute aortic dissection, and acute aortic endocarditis.

Aneurysmal Disease

The risk of rupture and dissection of the aortic root and ascending aorta is generally thought to be a function of size according to Laplace's Law, which states that wall tension in a cylinder is directly proportional to its diameter.[5] Much of what is known about the natural history of aneurysms according to size has been contributed by Elefteriades and his colleagues at Yale.[6,7] The risk of rupture or dissection increases dramatically once aneurysms approach 6 cm in diameter (**Fig. 2**). Based on these studies, the American College of Cardiology/American Heart Association guidelines state that in the absence of a connective tissue disorder or bicuspid aortic valve, that asymptomatic aneurysms of the ascending aorta should be electively repaired when they reach 5.5 cm diameter or if growth of 0.5 cm or more is documented on imaging studies over a period of 1 year.[8]

Patients with Marfan syndrome or other genetically mediated connective tissue disorders should undergo elective surgery at diameters of 4 to 5 cm depending on the condition. In patients with bicuspid aortic valve, elective surgery is recommended when the maximal diameter of the aortic root or ascending aorta approaches 5 cm. This also depends on the presence of significant aortic stenosis or regurgitation and the age and size of the patient. In a patient with an enlarged ascending aorta or aortic root undergoing cardiac surgery for other causes (coronary artery disease, cardiac valvular disease), most surgeons feel that the ascending aorta should be replaced if its diameter exceeds 4.5 cm. Because a single scale should not be applied to all patients regardless of their height or body habitus, the aortic size index was developed to predict the risk of rupture of a thoracic aortic aneurysm relative to the body surface area of a patient.[9] In fact, there are both electronic device applications and Web sites that allow physicians and patients to calculate their aortic size index, obesity controlled aortic size index, and cross-sectional area to height ratio to determine when elective surgery might be indicated.[10,11]

Patients with known aneurysms of the ascending aorta or aortic root that have not reached sufficient size for elective repair should be followed up regularly with either computed tomography or MRI to assess size and growth rate and echocardiography to determine aortic valve function. If the morphology of the aortic valve is not clear on 2-dimensional echocardiogram, transesophageal echocardiography is recommended to determine whether a patient has a bicuspid valve and to accurately assess the size and configuration of the aortic root. Aggressive blood pressure control with β-blockers, angiotensin-converting enzyme inhibitors, or angiotensin receptor blockers is essential in preventing rupture or dissection of aortic aneurysms. The authors recommend a target systolic blood pressure in the 120s mm Hg and carefully discuss activity limitations with patients who have aortic root or ascending aortic dilatation. These restrictions vary from relatively severe exercise limitations in patients with connective tissue disorders to carefully planned exercise regimens in those with bicuspid or tricuspid aortic valves. The authors have occasionally done exercise testing in these patients to determine their blood pressure response to exercise and to counsel them regarding acceptable blood pressure and heart rate with exercise. Pregnancy can be particularly risky for young women with bicuspid aortic valves and aortic root or ascending aortic dilatation.

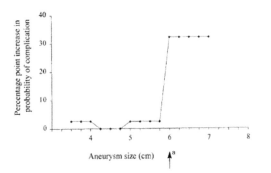

Fig. 2. Estimated effect of ascending aortic size on risk of complication. [a] Hinge point at 6.0 cm (*P*=.005). (*Adapted from* Coady MA, Rizzo JA, Hammond GI, et al. What is the appropriate size criterion for resection of thoracic aortic aneurysms? Thorac Cardiovasc Surg 1997;113(3):476–91; with permission.)

Acute Aortic Dissection

Acute aortic dissection involving the ascending aorta (Stanford Type A, DeBakey type I and II) has become one of the most common cardiac surgical emergencies. Failure to promptly diagnose and treat Stanford type A aortic dissection results in the death of the patient most of the time, usually within 48 hours. Aortic dissection requires aortic root replacement when the dissection tear extends below the sinotubular junction or if there is significant dilatation of the aortic root (>4.5 cm) with or without aortic valve regurgitation. Although most surgeons prefer an aortic valve conduit with reimplantation of the coronary arteries for aortic root replacement (modified Bentall procedure) in this scenario, some have reported excellent results with valve-sparing aortic root replacement.[12] If the dissection tear does not extend proximal to the sinotubular junction and there is no other aortic root condition, the ascending aorta can be replaced with a tube graft starting at the sinotubular junction without disturbing the aortic root. In experienced hands, aortic root replacement for type A aortic dissection can be performed with perioperative mortality rates of less than 15% and 5-year survival rates of 85%.[13]

Aortic Endocarditis

Infective endocarditis involving the aortic valve with abscess formation and aortic root destruction creates a serious surgical challenge. The goals of surgery for native or prosthetic aortic endocarditis are drainage of any abscess cavities, complete debridement of infected tissue, and aortic valve replacement without mechanical stress on the valvular suture line.[14] Many cardiac surgeons feel that aortic root reconstruction with a human homograft offers the best chance of treating the current infection and preventing recurrent endocarditis because it minimizes the amount of nonbiological material placed into the infected field when performing the aortic root reconstruction.[15] Others have found no difference in the rates of major complications or long-term survival between patients who received homograft root reconstruction for infective endocarditis and those who received either a mechanical or bioprosthetic valved conduit.[16]

The surgical treatment of prosthetic aortic endocarditis is even more complicated because of the added technical difficulty of working in a previously operated field filled with dense scar tissue. This treatment increases the risk of injury to surrounding structures, including the pulmonary artery, left atrium, right ventricle, and the coronary arteries. Wilbring and colleagues[17] reported a series of aortic root operations for prosthetic endocarditis with a perioperative mortality rate of 12.9% and a 5-year survival rate of 75.3%. The

most common cause of death was septic multiorgan failure in 42.9% of deaths.[17]

SURGICAL PROCEDURES FOR AORTIC ROOT DISEASE

Surgical procedures that replace or reconstruct the aortic root are technically more demanding than simple aortic valve replacement or aortic valve replacement plus replacement of the ascending aorta. The requirement for dissection and reimplantation of the coronary arteries adds an increased risk of coronary artery injury or distortion that can result in bleeding or cardiac ischemic complications. Furthermore, the aortic root and coronary artery ostia are particularly fragile in patients with connective tissue disorders such as Marfan syndrome or in patients with acute Stanford type A aortic dissection who require aortic root replacement. Surgical dissection of the base of the aortic root for valve-sparing procedures can be complicated by injury to adjacent structures requiring repair. These structures include the pulmonary artery, right ventricular outflow tract, and the right and left atria. As such, aortic root surgery should be performed by surgeons with specialized training and experience with these demanding operations. These surgeons are not ubiquitous. In fact, a recent inquiry of the Society of Thoracic Surgeons National Cardiac Surgery database found that the median yearly number of aortic root procedures performed was 2 per center, with only 5% of centers reporting more than 16 aortic root procedures per year.[18]

The decision regarding the most suitable aortic root procedure for a given patient depends on his or her underlying age, diagnosis, and the condition of the aortic valve. In addition to total aortic root replacement with replacement of the aortic valve with a mechanical or bioprosthesis, aortic valve-sparing procedures have recently become popular for patients with structurally intact aortic valves. Whereas the aortic valve can be spared in many patients with moderate or even severe aortic insufficiency, a functional and long-lasting valve repair is unlikely in patients who have aortic valves that are calcified or significantly striated.

Total Aortic Root Replacement

Depending on the circumstances, the aortic root can be replaced with a Dacron valved conduit, a cadaveric human aortic homograft, or a pulmonary artery autograft.

Replacement of the aortic root with a Dacron conduit and aortic valve prosthesis was first described in 1968 by Bentall and Debono at the

Hammersmith Hospital in London.[19] Because of the porous nature of Dacron grafts available at the time, hemorrhage was the most feared early complication of these procedures. To control bleeding from the Dacron graft, the aneurysm sac was wrapped around it and a saphenous vein fistula created from the peri-graft space to the right atrium to shunt shed blood back into the heart. The modern aortic root replacement usually consists of replacing the aortic valve and root with an albumin-impregnated Dacron conduit for better hemostasis, containing either a mechanical or bioprosthetic aortic valve (bioroot). These valved conduits are commercially available in many sizes, frequently with the valve already attached to the Dacron graft. The coronary ostia are reimplanted directly into the Dacron graft (**Fig. 3**).

Aortic root replacement (modified Bentall procedure) is most commonly performed in patients with aneurysmal disease of the aortic root or patients with acute aortic dissection in which the intimal tear extends below the sinotubular junction. When performed electively on patients with aortic root aneurysm, results are excellent with perioperative mortality rates of less than 4%.[20]

Cadaveric Human Homograft

Human aortic homografts were first implanted by Ross in 1962 and were popularized for aortic root

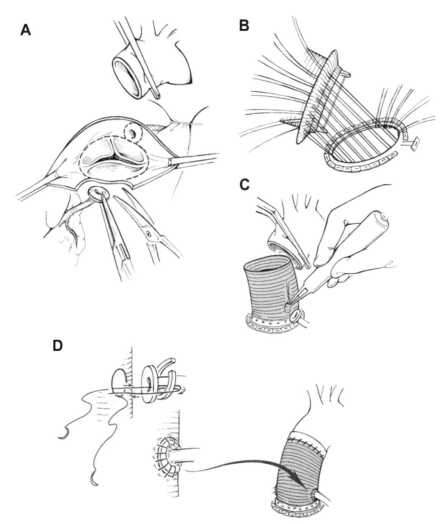

Fig. 3. The modified Bentall procedures. (*A*) After resecting the aneurysmal tissue, the coronary buttons are carefully dissected for reimplantation. (*B*) A valved conduit is sutured to the aortic annulus. (*C*) Openings are created in the graft for implantation of the coronary buttons. (*D*) Coronary buttons anastomosed to the Dacron graft. (*Adapted from* Parsa CJ, Hughes GC. Surgical options to content with thoracic aortic pathology. Semin Roentgenol 2009;44(1):29–51; with permission.)

reconstruction in the 1980s (**Fig. 4**).[21,22] In addition to not requiring anticoagulation, they have excellent hemodynamic performance and are thought to be resistant to infection. It was initially proposed that homografts might offer improved durability over stented bioprosthetic valves in younger patients who wanted to avoid the lifelong anticoagulation associated with mechanical prosthetic aortic valves. However, aortic homografts deteriorate over time at a variable rate depending on the patient's age, source of the homograft, and the sterilization and preservation methods.[23,24] Cryopreserved cadaveric human aortic homografts are the most popular type of commercially available aortic allograft. However, their limited availability and need for specialized storage, technical complexity of implantation, and tendency to calcify and degenerate over time have limited their clinical utility. Although controversial, many feel that they are the valve conduit of choice in patients with infective endocarditis and significant periannular abscess. In fact, the Society of Thoracic Surgeons guidelines for the surgical treatment of aortic valve disease state that there is class 1 evidence to suggest that homograft replacement of the aortic valve should be considered for patients with extensive active endocarditis with destruction of the aortic annulus (level of evidence B). Furthermore, for patients undergoing homograft replacement of the aortic valve, a total root replacement technique is recommended.[25]

Pulmonary Autograft for Aortic Root Replacement (The Ross Procedure)

Aortic root replacement with an autologous pulmonary autograft was first described by Donald Ross in 1967.[26] The Ross procedure subsequently became a popular option for replacing the aortic valve in the pediatric population

because the native pulmonary valve functions well in the aortic position, does not require anticoagulation, and seems to grow with the growth of the young patient. Furthermore, the durability of the pulmonary root in the aortic position can be excellent, especially if the aortic annulus is reinforced at the time of surgery.[27] The Ross procedure is technically intricate. The aortic root is dissected and coronary artery ostia prepared for reimplantation similar to a homograft or valved conduit root replacement. The pulmonary artery is then harvested without injury to it or the surrounding structures. This harvest includes great care not to injure the left main coronary artery as it courses behind the pulmonary artery trunk. The pulmonary autograft is then anastomosed to the aortic annulus and the coronary arteries reimplanted followed by reconstruction of the pulmonary outflow tract with a cadaveric homograft (**Fig. 5**).

Although use of the Ross procedure has been extended by some surgeons to a select group of adults, most feel that its greatest utility lies in the pediatric population and young adults.[28] This use is justified by the technical demands of aortic and pulmonary artery reconstruction and the excellent results afforded by other aortic root operations in the adult population.

Valve-Sparing Aortic Root Replacement

In 1992, Tirone David and the Toronto group[29,30] coined the term *aortic valve-sparing* operations to describe conservative procedures on the aortic valve in patients with aortic root aneurysms. They then went on to classify valve-sparing operations into aortic valve reimplantation and aortic root remodeling.[31] The remodeling operation was championed by Sarsam and Yacoub[32] and involves replacement of the sinus segments with a scalloped polyester graft. In the reimplantation procedure, the aortic valve and commissures are sewn into a Dacron tube graft, creating neosinuses of Valsalva in between the commissures. The coronary arteries are then implanted into the new sinuses. Several refinements to this operation, now dubbed the David V, were aimed at preventing dilatation of the aortic annulus with recurrent aortic insufficiency over time. There have also been modifications suggested from other centers.[33]

Although a technically more difficult operation than aortic root replacement with a commercial valved conduit, the early and long-term results of the valve-sparing reimplantation technique have been excellent for patients with both bicuspid and tricuspid valves, including patients

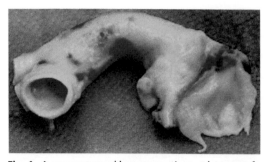

Fig. 4. A cryopreserved human aortic root homograft. (*From* Peng YG, Martin T, Horowitz T, et al. Repair of concomitant valvular endocarditis using a single homograft. Ann Thorac Surg 2009;88(2):e14–5; with permission.)

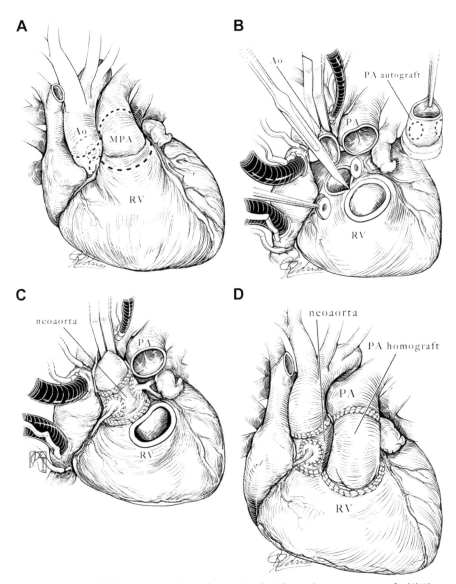

Fig. 5. The Ross procedure. (*A*) The aortic root is to be replaced with a pulmonary autograft. (*B*) The aortic valve and root are resected, preparing the coronary buttons for reimplantation. The pulmonary autograft is harvested. (*C*) The aortic root is reconstructed using the pulmonary autograft. (*D*) The pulmonary valve and trunk are replaced with a cadaveric PA or aortic homograft. (*Adapted from* Mavroudis C, Backer CL, Kaushal S. Aortic stenosis and aortic insufficiency in children: impact of valvuloplasty and modified ross-konno procedure. Semin Thorac Cardiovasc Surg Pediatr Card Surg Annu 2009;12(1):76–86; with permission.)

with connective tissue disorders such as Marfan syndrome.[34,35] Valve-sparing operations are particularly attractive for younger patients because concern of structural valve deterioration from a stented bioprosthetic valve is eliminated as is the need for chronic anticoagulation. The indications for these operations are expanding; some surgeons have expanded the use of the valve-sparing reimplantation technique to patients with acute aortic dissection requiring root replacement.[12]

SUMMARY

An increased understanding of the anatomy and pathophysiology of the aortic root has led to the development of several surgical procedures designed to replace the root for aneurysmal disease, acute aortic dissection, and infective endocarditis. In experienced hands, these operations can be safely performed with excellent early and late results. Many patients, including those with bicuspid aortic valves and connective tissue disorders, are candidates for valve-sparing operations that appear to be associated with excellent long-term results without the need for anticoagulation.

REFERENCES

1. Yankah CA, Pasic M, Ivanitskaia-Kühn E, et al. The aortic root. In: Yankah CA, Weng Y, Hetzer R, editors. Berlin: Springer-Verlag; 2010. p. 13–21.
2. Leonardo da Vinci. Anatomical drawings from the Royal collections. London: The Royal Academy of Arts; 1977. p. 35A.
3. Valsalva AM. Arteria magnae sinus. In: Morgagni JB, editor. Opera. Venice: Apud Franciscum Pitteri; 1740. p. 1–129.
4. David T. The role of aortic root disease. Implications for treatment of aortic stenois and regurgitation. Postgraduate course. The 2005 AATS meeting was held in Moscone West Convention Center. San Francisco, April 10–13, 2005.
5. Basford JR. The law of Laplace and its relevance to contemporary medicine and rehabilitation. Arch Phys Med Rehabil 2002;83:1165–70.
6. Coady MA, Rizzo JA, Hammond GL, et al. What is the appropriate size criterion for resection of thoracic aortic aneurysms? J Thorac Cardiovasc Surg 1997;113:476–911.
7. Davies RR, Goldstein LJ, Coady MA, et al. Yearly rupture or dissection rates for thoracic aortic aneurysms: simple prediction based on size. Ann Thorac Surg 2002;73:17–28.
8. Hiratzka LF, Bakris GL, Beckman JA, et al. 2010 ACCF/AHA/AATS/ACR/ASA/SCA/SCAI/SIR/STS/SVM guidelines for the diagnosis and management of patients with Thoracic Aortic Disease. Circulation 2010; 122(4):e410.
9. Davies RR, Gallo A, Coady MA, et al. Novel measurement of relative aortic size predicts rupture of thoracic aortic aneurysms. Ann Thorac Surg 2006;81:169–77.
10. Available at: Valleyheartandvascular.com.
11. AORTA: Aortic surgery guidelines electronic device app. Sponsored by Montreal Heart Institute.
12. Leshnower BG, Myng RJ, McPherson L, et al. Midterm results of David V valve-sparing aortic root replacement in acute type a aortic dissection. Ann Thorac Surg 2015;99(3):795–800 [discussion: 800–1].
13. Nishida H, Tabata M, Fukui T, et al. Surgical strategy and outcome for aortic root in patients undergoing repair of acute type a aortic dissection. Ann Thorac Surg 2016;101(4):1464–9.
14. Smail H, Pankaj S, Zimmet A, et al. Reconstruction and replacement of the aortic root in destructive endocarditis. Oper Tech Thorac Cardiovasc Surg 2016;20:336–54.
15. Niwaya K, Knott-Craig CJ, Santangelo K, et al. Advantage of autograft and homograft valve replacement for complex aortic valve endocarditis. Ann Thorac Surg 1999;67:1603–8.
16. Jassar AS, Bavaria JE, Szeto WY, et al. Graft selection for aortic root replacement in complex active endocarditis: does it matter? Ann Thorac Surg 2012; 93:480–8.
17. Wilbring M, Tugtekin SM, Alexiou K, et al. Composite aortic root replacement for complex prosthetic valve endocarditis. Initial clinical results and long-term follow-up of high-risk patients. Ann Thorac Surg 2012;94:1967–74.
18. Stamou SC, Williams ML, Gunn TM, et al. Aortic root surgery in the United States: a report of the Society of Thoracic Surgeons database. J Thorac Cardiovasc Surg 2015;149:116–22.
19. Bentall H, DeBono A. A technique for complete replacement of the ascending aorta. Thorax 1968; 23:338–433.
20. Etz CD, von Asperm K, Girrbach FF, et al. Long-term survival after composite mechanical aortic root replacement: a consecutive series of 448 cases. J Thorac Cardiovasc Surg 2013;145:S41–7.
21. Hopkins RA. Cardiac reconstructions with allograft valves. New York: Springer-Verlag; 1989.
22. Ross DN. Homograft replacement of the aortic valve. Lancet 1962;2:487.
23. O'Brien MF, McGiffin DC, Stafford EG, et al. Allograft aortic valve replacement: longterm comparative clinical analysis of viable cryopreserved and antibiotic stored 4 8C stored valves. J Card Surg 1991;6:534–43.
24. Lund O, Chandrasekaran V, Grocott-Mason R, et al. Primary aortic valve replacementwith allografts over twenty-five years: valve-related and procedure-related determinants of outcome. J Thorac Cardiovasc Surg 1999;117(1):77–90.
25. Svensson LG, Adams DH, Bonow RO, et al. Aortic valve and ascending aorta guidelines for management and quality measures. Ann Thorac Surg 2013;95:1–66.
26. Ross DN. Replacement of aortic and mitral valves with a pulmonary autograft. Lancet 1967;2:956–8.
27. Kallio M, Pihkala J, Sairanen H, et al. Long term results of the Ross procedure in a population-based followup. Eur J Cardiothorac Surg 2015;47:e164–70.
28. Bansal N, Ram Kumar S, Baker CJ, et al. Age related outcomes of the Ross procedure over 20 years. Ann Thorac Surg 2015;99:2077–85.
29. David T. Aortic valve repair and aortic valve-sparing operations. Invite commentary. J Thorac Cardiovasc Surg 2015;149:9–11.
30. David TE, Feindel CM. An aorticvalve–sparingoperationforpatientswithaortic incompetence and aneurysm of the ascending aorta. J Thorac Cardiovasc Surg 1992;103:617–21 [discussion: 622].
31. David TE, Feindel CM, Bos J. Repair of the aortic valve in patients with aortic insufficiency and aortic

root aneurysm. J Thorac Cardiovasc Surg 1995;109: 345–51 [discussion: 351–2].

32. Sarsam MA, Yacoub M. Remodeling of the aortic valve anulus. J Thorac Cardiovasc Surg 1993;105: 435–8.

33. Miller DC. Rationale and results of the Stanford modification of the David V reimplantation technique for valve-sparing aortic root replacement. J Thorac Cardiovasc Surg 2015;149:S18–20.

34. Richardt D, Stierle U, Sievers HH. Long-term results after aortic valve-sparing-reimplantation operation (David) in bicuspid aortic valve. J Heart Valve Dis 2015;24(1):4–9.

35. Yamauchi AM, Taketani MT, Shimada S, et al. Long-term outcome after the original and simple modified technique of valve-sparing aortic root reimplantation in Marfan based population, David V Unversity of Tokyo modification. J Cardiol 2016;67(1):86–91.

Acute Type A Aortic Dissection

Ramsey S. Elsayed, MD, Robbin G. Cohen, MD, MMM, Fernando Fleischman, MD,
Michael E. Bowdish, MD*

KEYWORDS

- Cardiac surgery • Aortic dissection • Diagnosis • Management • Outcomes

KEY POINTS

- Type A aortic dissection occurs when an intimal tear in the aorta creates a false lumen in the ascending aorta.
- Type A aortic dissection is a surgical emergency requiring prompt diagnosis and treatment.
- Computed tomographic angiogram is the diagnostic modality of choice.
- Repair involves replacement of the ascending aorta with or without aortic root and/or arch replacement.
- Contemporary in-hospital mortality is 10% to 15% but is highly related to comorbidities, extent of repair needed, and postoperative complications.

INTRODUCTION AND ANATOMY

The aorta is a conduit that extends from the left ventricle that delivers pulsatile blood distally to organs and tissue beds. Acute dissection of the ascending aorta is a lethal disease that requires prompt diagnosis and surgical intervention. Once almost exclusively a postmortem diagnosis, improvements in the accuracy of diagnostic modalities, anesthetic techniques, extracorporeal perfusion, methods of end organ protection during aortic replacement, types of prosthetic grafts, surgical techniques, and critical care have markedly improved outcomes over the last 40 years.[1]

It is useful to understand the anatomy of the aorta in order to appreciate the complexity of acute aortic syndromes (**Fig. 1**A). The annulus, aortic valvular leaflets, and coronary arteries along with the sinus of Valsalva comprise the aortic root (**Fig. 1**B). It is followed anatomically by the ascending aorta, which extends from the sinotubular junction to the innominate artery. The aortic arch, where supra-aortic branches arise, extends from the innominate artery to the left subclavian artery. The descending thoracic aorta, where numerous intercostal arteries arise, extends from the left subclavian artery to the level of the diaphragm. Finally, the abdominal aorta is defined by the length of the aorta below the diaphragm down to the iliac bifurcation.

It is also important to differentiate the terms aneurysm, pseudoaneurysm, and dissection. An aortic aneurysm, also referred to as a "true aneurysm," is a full-thickness dilatation of all the aortic wall layers (intima, media, and adventitia). If left untreated, the aortic wall continues to weaken and becomes unable to withstand the forces of luminal blood pressure, leading to progressive dilatation and rupture which usually occurs in the presence of one or more synergistic risk factors, such as male sex, smoking, hypertension, and atherosclerosis.[2] On the other hand, a pseudoaneurysm, also

Disclosure Statement: No authors have a relationship with a commercial entity with a direct financial interest in the subject matter or materials discussed in this article.
Department of Surgery, Keck School of Medicine of USC, University of Southern California, 1520 San Pablo Street, HCC II, Suite 4300, Los Angeles, CA 90033, USA
* Corresponding author.
E-mail address: Michael.Bowdish@med.usc.edu

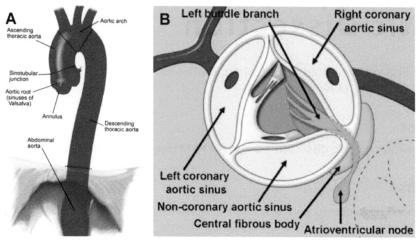

Fig. 1. (A) Anatomic classification of the aorta. (B) Anatomy of the aortic root. (*From* [A] Ladich E, Butany J, Virmani R. Chapter 5: Aneurysms of the aorta: ascending, thoracic and abdominal and their management. In: Butany J, Buja ML, editors. Cardiovascular pathology. 4th edition. Philadelphia: Elsevier; 2016, p. 170; and [B] Tran PK, Tsang V. When and how to enlarge the small aortic root. Semin Thorac Cardiovasc Surg Pediatr Card Surg Annu 2016;19(1):56; with permission.)

referred to as a "false aneurysm," is a dilatation in the partial thickness of the aortic wall. It usually results from a traumatic tear or an acute infection in the aortic wall but is contained by the surrounding tissue. Pseudoaneurysms might be caused by penetrating or blunt trauma, acute mycotic processes, or iatrogenically during cardiac catheterization or after cardiac surgery.[3,4]

Dissection of the aorta occurs when there is separation of the aortic media. It is typically caused by pulsatile blood flow from a tear in the intimal layer of the aortic wall, exposing the underlying media to the driving force of blood and thus creating a parallel "false lumen" in the aortic wall. The alternative, less common mechanism is from bleeding within the aortic wall, commonly referred to as an aortic intramural hematoma. Regardless of the site of origin or mechanism, the dissection plane can then propagate to extend from the aortic root to any or all of the distal aortic branches due to the persistent intraluminal pressure. Although somewhat controversial, it is the authors' opinion that an intramural hematoma is no different than a dissection caused by an intimal tear and should be afforded the same treatment and urgency when located in the ascending aorta.

CLASSIFICATION

Two classification systems for aortic dissections are commonly used (**Fig. 2**). The Stanford classification system is most commonly used and has gained widespread acceptance since its initial introduction in 1970. If the dissection involves the ascending aorta, it is a Stanford type A. If the

ascending aorta proximal to the innominate artery is not involved in the process, the dissection is called a Stanford type B. The less commonly used DeBakey classification system was initially proposed in 1955 and then modified in 1965 and 1982 to correspond more closely with the Stanford classification system based on whether the ascending aorta was involved regardless of the site of the intimal tear or distal extent of the dissection.[5,6] DeBakey type I and II dissections both involve the ascending aorta; however, a type I extends beyond the innominate artery, whereas a type II is confined to the ascending aorta. DeBakey type I and II dissections both correspond to a Stanford type A dissection. A DeBakey type III dissection corresponds to a Stanford type B dissection, where the ascending aorta proximal to the innominate artery is not involved.

EPIDEMIOLOGY AND PATHOPHYSIOLOGY

Aortic dissection is the most common and disastrous event to affect the aorta. It occurs nearly 3 times as frequently as rupture of abdominal aortic aneurysms in the United States.[7] Studies of acute aortic syndromes recorded at tertiary care centers suggest that type A aortic dissection remains the most frequently transferred emergency through regional rapid transport systems.[8,9] It occurs with a greater frequency than type B aortic dissections, while both types occur more frequently in men in the sixth decade of life.[10,11] Women with aortic dissection are more likely to present at an older age than men and to have atypical symptoms, which often delays the diagnosis and subsequent

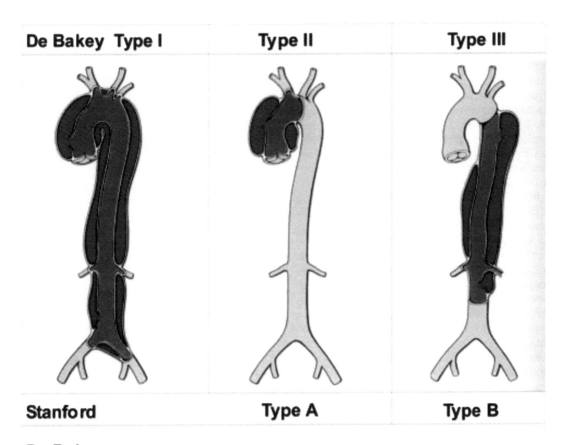

De Bakey

Type I   Originates in the ascending aorta, propagates at least to the aortic arch and often beyond it distally

Type II   Originates in and is confined to the ascending aorta

Type III   Originates in the descending aorta and extends distally down the aorta or, rarely, retrograde into the aortic arch and ascending aorta

Stanford

Type A   All dissections involving the ascending aorta, regardless of the site of origin

Type B   All dissections not involving the ascending aorta

Fig. 2. Stanford and Debakey classification systems of thoracic aortic dissection. (*From* Mukherjee D, Eagle KA. Aortic dissection—an update. Curr Probl Cardiol 2005;30(6):293; with permission.)

treatment, leading to higher mortality in some studies. The International Registry for Aortic Dissection has shown that patients with aortic dissections who are of African descent present at a younger age and with a higher incidence of cocaine abuse, hypertension, and diabetes than white patients.[12]

The pathogenesis of aortic dissection remains controversial. Over the years, several hypotheses have been elucidated regarding the explanation behind the intimal disruption that allows blood flow to create a false lumen within the media of the aorta.[13] Of note, shear forces may lead to further tears in the intimal flap, which can produce exit sites or additional entry sites for blood flow into the false lumen. Whether due to an inherent instability of the aortic wall as in congenital connective tissue diseases or to acquired conditions such as atherosclerotic degeneration due to aging, compromise in the aortic wall remains the fundamental component of the abnormality of aortic dissection. In a minority of patients, mostly children, biochemical abnormalities within the medial layer on which normal mechanical forces act to create the intimal tear remained suspect, although the link between the abnormal media, termed cystic medial degeneration, and the primary tear has not been properly established.[14] Alternatively, data have been published supporting the relationship between aortic dissection and intramural hematoma. It has been suggested that bleeding from the vasa vasorum into the media creates a mass effect, which, in turn, creates numerous areas of increased stress in the intima during the diastolic phase, which weakens the inner aortic wall and permits intimal disruption.[15] This phenomena exists in 10% to 20% of patients with type A aortic dissection and is thought to be a precursor for its development. In addition, penetrating atherosclerotic aortic ulcers have also been implicated as a source of intimal disruption; therefore, most institutions treat penetrating atherosclerotic ulcers of the ascending aorta similarly to true type A aortic dissection.[16–18]

The primary tear in type A aortic dissection is usually located on the right anterior aspect of the ascending aorta, spiraling around the arch into the descending thoracic and abdominal aorta on the left and posteriorly. Furthermore, dissections may extend in a retrograde fashion involving the coronary ostia; this occurs in roughly 6% to 11% of dissections.[19,20] The main cause of death is due to myocardial ischemia or aortic rupture into the pericardium, which occurs in about 80% of deaths from acute type A aortic dissection.[21]

RISK FACTORS

Although no single disorder is responsible for aortic dissection, several risk factors have been identified that could damage the aortic wall and lead to dissection (**Box 1**).[2,22]

Cardiovascular

As mentioned earlier, atherosclerotic degeneration of the aorta is a common predisposing factor to aortic dissection, leading to instability of the aortic wall, which includes intimal thickening, fibrosis, calcification, extracellular fatty acid deposition, and extracellular matrix degradation that compromise the elastic properties of the wall.[2] It should be noted that atherosclerosis is only a risk factor for aortic dissection in the setting of preexisting aneurysms or in the case of atherosclerotic ulceration.[23,24] Older age, smoking, cocaine

---

Box 1
Risk factors for aortic dissection

Lifestyle and cardiovascular risk factors
- Long-term hypertension
- Old age
- Dyslipidemia
- Pregnancy-induced hypervolemia
- Weight-lifting
- Smoking
- Cocaine abuse

Congenital and connective tissue disorders
- Bicuspid aortic valve
- Marfan syndrome
- Loeys-Dietz syndrome
- Ehlers-Danlos syndrome
- Turner syndrome

Trauma
- Aortic transection
  - Motor vehicle deceleration injury
  - Falling from height

Iatrogenic
- Cardiac catheterization
- Arterial cannulation for cardiopulmonary bypass
- Aortic cross-clamping during valvular or aortic surgery
- Intra-aortic balloon pumps

Vascular inflammation
- Autoimmune disease
  - Giant cell arteritis
  - Takayasu arteritis
  - Bechet disease
- Infectious disease
  - Syphilis
  - Tuberculosis

Aortic aneurysm

---

abuse, dyslipidemia, and increased levels of apolipoprotein A1 are dissection promoters but usually act as synergistic factors.

Hypertension is the mechanical force most often associated with dissection and is found in greater than 80% of cases[25]; it contributes to the production of proinflammatory cytokines and matrix metalloproteinases and leads to excessive extracellular matrix degradation.[26] Similarly, hypervolemia, high cardiac output, and an abnormal hormonal setting contribute to the increased incidence in pregnancy, but the mechanism remains unclear.[27,28]

Connective Tissue Disease

Mutations in various connective tissue genes predispose individuals to aortic dissection.[29] Marfan syndrome, Loeys-Dietz syndrome, Ehler-Danlos syndrome, and Turner syndrome are the most common genetic disorders associated with aortic dissection.

Marfan syndrome
Approximately 5% of patients with aortic dissection have Marfan syndrome, which is an autosomal dominant disorder caused by a mutation in the FBN1 gene, which encodes fibrillin 1, a component of elastin-associated microfibrils that are located mainly in the media. FBN1 mutation results in a predisposition for the development of aortic aneurysms and dissections as well as skeletal and ocular features.[30]

Loeys-Dietz syndrome
Loeys-Dietz syndrome is similar to Marfan syndrome, an autosomal dominant disorder caused by a mutation in the TGFB1 or TGFB2, which encode transforming growth factor-β receptors. Patients carrying this mutation suffer aneurysms and dissections in other arteries as well as the aorta.[30]

Ehler-Danlos syndrome
A mutation in the COL3A1 gene that encodes type III collagen is responsible for the vascular form of Ehler-Danlos syndrome. This type is associated with distinct facial features, easy bruising, thin hyperextensible skin, and rupture of uterus, intestines, or arteries. Median survival is 48 years with most deaths due to thoracic or abdominal dissection.[31,32]

Turner syndrome
Turner syndrome is characterized by the absence of an X chromosome in an otherwise phenotypic woman (45 + XO). Bicuspid aortic valves and preductal aortic coarctation are the most common cardiac abnormalities seen in Turner syndrome, while aortic dissection is the most common aortic disease and is 6 times more common in Turner syndrome than in the general population, with an estimated incidence of 40 cases per 100,000 Turner syndrome–years.[33,34] These patients are characterized by short stature, a broad chest, and horseshoe kidneys. Current US guidance suggests that children and adolescents with this syndrome should have a full evaluation with thoracic MRI at an age when it can be performed without sedation.[35]

Trauma

Transection of the aorta as a result of trauma rarely can occur at the aortic isthmus, sinotubular junction, or distal aortic arch, which are considered the "fixed points" of the aorta susceptible to transection in the event of blunt trauma (eg, rapid deceleration injury in a motor vehicle accident).[36] Although true traumatic dissection is uncommon, it can occur.

Iatrogenic

Iatrogenic dissection of the aortic intima may be caused by central and femoral cannulation for cardiopulmonary bypass, aortic cross-clamping, and intra-aortic balloon pumps. Cardiac catheterization procedures such as percutaneous coronary interventions may also result in dissection.[37]

Vascular Inflammation

Particular autoimmune and infectious diseases have been implicated in the development of aortic dissection. Persistence of aortic inflammation along with changes in the degree of elasticity of the aortic media greatly contributes to the risk of intimal disruption in association with one or more of the previously described factors. Giant cell arteritis, Takayasu arteritis, and Bechet disease are the most common autoimmune diseases, whereas syphilis and tuberculosis are the most common infectious diseases associated with aortic dissection.[38,39]

Aortic Aneurysm

Thoracic aortic aneurysms are associated with increased risk of dissection at the level of the diseased segment. Aneurysms with a diameter greater than 5.5 mm, yearly growth rate greater than 0.5 mm, or symptomatic should undergo evaluation for surgical repair.[40] Old age and longstanding hypertension are thought to be influential on the association between increased aneurysm size and increased risk of rupture or dissection.[41,42]

CLINICAL PRESENTATION

Immediate death following a short period of symptoms or no symptoms occurs in an overwhelmingly high percentage of patients with acute aortic dissection. Some investigators report the immediate mortality to be as high as 40%.[43] Mortality results from aortic rupture, pericardial tamponade leading to cardiogenic shock, acute aortic valve regurgitation, and acute myocardial ischemia in the case of coronary ostia involvement.

The diagnosis of acute type A aortic dissection requires a high index of suspicion. Up to 30% of patients are initially misdiagnosed.[44] The extent of dissection, hemodynamic stability, presence or absence of malperfusion, and prompt surgical intervention are the main determinants of clinical outcomes. Type A aortic dissection patients are usually younger than their type B aortic dissection counterparts, although type A aortic dissection is not uncommon in older patients with multiple coexisting medical conditions.

In-depth history taking and a detailed physical examination are essential in the diagnosis of type A aortic dissection. A high index of suspicion is warranted in the setting of severe "ripping" or "tearing" retrosternal or substernal chest pain. In the International Registry of Aortic Dissection, the sudden onset chest pain was the presenting symptom in 85% of patients.[45] This pain is due to aortic adventitial nerve fibers being stretched by the dissection itself. It is important to mention that the location of maximum pain might change as the dissection extends in a retrograde or antegrade fashion. This pain may disappear spontaneously or after the institution of medical therapy, however. Although most patients with type A aortic dissection present with pain, painless dissection may also occur.

As many as 33% of acute type A aortic dissection patients present with symptoms of end organ malperfusion, which substantially impacts outcomes. Cerebral, peripheral, and visceral malperfusion can occur separately or in combination and have been shown to be independent predictors of postoperative outcomes.[46]

The presentation of acute type A aortic dissection with stroke, paraplegia, renal failure, abdominal pain, or a compromised lower extremity elucidates the involvement of the brachiocephalic, intercostal or lumbar, renal, mesenteric vessels, or iliac vessels. On physical examination, the absence of upper extremity pulses suggests ascending aortic involvement, whereas faint or nonpalpable lower extremity pulses indicate the extension of the dissection beyond the iliac arteries. In addition, cardiac tamponade should be suspected in the presence of Beck triad, acute aortic regurgitation in the presence of a diastolic murmur, or an S3 on auscultation, and hemothorax due to aortic leak should be considered in the case of unilateral loss of breath sounds.

Other rare symptoms include hoarseness of voice, upper airway obstruction, rupture into the tracheobronchial tree with hemoptysis, rupture into the esophagus with hematemesis, dysphagia, superior vena cava syndrome, pulsating neck masses, Horner syndrome, or the presence of a continuous murmur that might indicate rupture of the dissection into the atria or left ventricle with secondary congestive heart failure.

DIAGNOSIS

Expeditious diagnosis and a high level of clinical suspicion of type A aortic dissection are required to optimize outcomes. Routine diagnostic studies should be obtained: blood tests including cardiac enzymes to rule out a myocardial infarction, an electrocardiogram (ECG), and a chest radiograph, but are seldom sufficient to confirm the diagnosis.

Advances in noninvasive imaging have aided the diagnosis of type A aortic dissection. Historically diagnosed primarily by aortography, computed tomography angiography (CTA) is the current preferred diagnostic modality.

Computed Tomography

CTA is noninvasive, easy to perform, readily available, quick, and relatively inexpensive. The visualization of 2 distinct lumens in the ascending aorta divided by an intimal flap establishes the diagnosis of type A aortic dissection (**Fig. 3**). In addition to establishing the diagnosis, information as to the location of the intimal tear, extent of dissection, and status of arch vessels is also provided, which assists in surgical planning. If the heart rate is well controlled, ECG-gated CTA can also be used to visualize the coronary vasculature.[47] The sensitivity and specificity of this imaging modality approach 100% (82%-100% and 90%-100%, respectively). Despite these numerous benefits, it is not without limitations. It must be used with caution in patients with renal failure or uncontrolled diabetes because iodinated contrast might worsen kidney function; moreover, it is contraindicated in patients with a history of allergy to iodinated dye.

Transesophageal Echocardiography

Because of the anatomic proximity of the esophagus to the aorta, transesophageal echocardiography (TEE) is very useful for obtaining high-resolution real-time images of the aorta. It is especially useful in demonstrating the presence of a true and false lumen as well as providing information about ventricular and aortic valve function. TEE is especially useful in patients wherein contrast is absolutely contraindicated. The sensitivity of TEE in acute type A aortic dissection approaches 100% with a lesser specificity of 70% to 100% due to reverberation artifacts.[48] TEE is less useful for

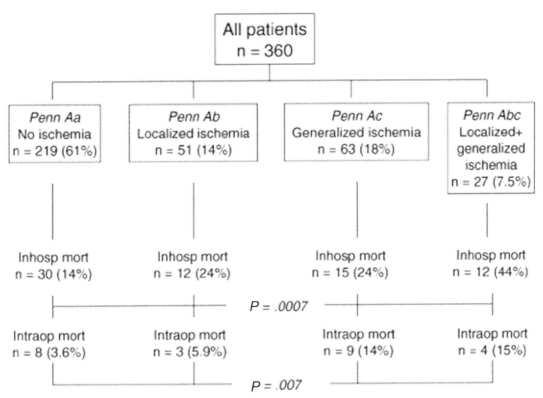

Fig. 3. Distribution of preoperative ischemia complications according to the Penn classification, with corresponding in-hospital (Inhosp mort) and intraoperative (Intraop mort) mortality. (*From* Olsson C, Hillebrant CG, Liska J, et al. Mortality in acute type A aortic dissection: validation of the Penn classification. Ann Thorac Surg 2011;92(4):1380; with permission.)

the definitive diagnosis of acute type A aortic dissection.[49]

MRI

The use of MRI in the diagnosis of acute type A aortic dissection is limited because it is not as readily available as CTA and is time consuming, although it can definitely be diagnostic and provide all the information needed to plan operative repair. MRI is more useful to assess aortic remodeling in patients with previous aortic repairs who have renal disease.

INITIAL MANAGEMENT

There is no role for preoperative stabilization once a diagnosis of type A aortic dissection has been established. After confirming the diagnosis, the patient is ideally transferred directly to the operating room for operative repair (**Fig. 4**). If the patient is at a center without operative capabilities, aggressive blood pressure control should be initiated, and the prompt transfer to a center with aortic expertise arranged. Systolic blood pressure should be maintained at less than 100 mm Hg to

reduce the sheer force within the aorta. Intravenous beta-blockers (esmolol, labetalol, or propranolol) are considered first-line therapy, followed by nipride or nitroprusside. Calcium-channel blockers can be substituted in lieu of beta-blockers in the presence of asthma or other contraindications.

Continuous neurologic status as well as blood pressure and urine output monitoring is imperative. Insertion of arterial, venous, and urinary catheters is mandatory, but should not delay transfer to the operating room.

Although open surgical repair is recommended for acute type A aortic dissection, there are some patients in which repair is futile. Those presenting with severe neurologic deficits, advanced debilitating systemic diseases that limit life expectancy, extreme frailty, and advanced age (>80 years) generally have extremely poor outcomes. Those presenting with abdominal ischemia should also be approached with caution with consideration for initial laparotomy before type A repair. The authors have found that very few patients who present with abdominal ischemia survive.

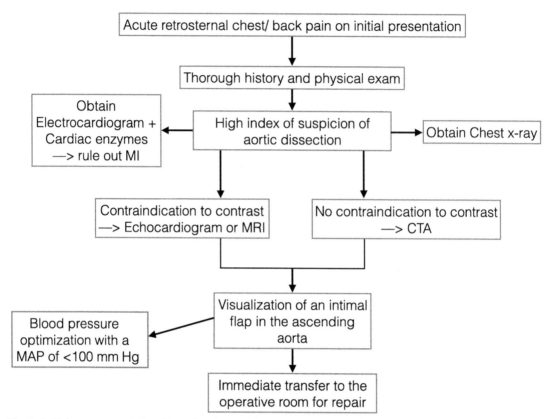

Fig. 4. Initial management algorithm of patients with acute type A aortic dissection. MAP, mean arterial pressure; MI, myocardial infarction.

SURGICAL MANAGEMENT

The essential principles of surgical repair of type A aortic dissection are to protect the patient's heart and brain, and to resect, at a minimum, the portion of the aorta with the intimal tear, and obliterate the false lumen of the dissected aorta. The authors' approach to type A aortic dissection repair has been described previously.[50] These operations are difficult and can tax even the master surgeon, especially because they are emergencies, require complex surgical decision making, and are technically demanding. Acute aortic dissection repair can necessitate a variety of operations, from simple replacement of the ascending aorta to aortic root replacement and/or a version of total arch replacement. Although there are differing opinions regarding what constitutes the optimal repair of the acutely dissected aorta, the authors' approach is to always replace the entire ascending aorta and to selectively replace the aortic root or arch based on the presence or absence of intimal tears or other abnormality. In this approach, the authors always address the ascending aorta, but only intervene on the more complex aortic root or arch when necessary to preserve life.

Different approaches exist to provide cerebral protection during operative repair: deep hypothermic circulatory arrest, retrograde cerebral perfusion, and antegrade cerebral perfusion are the most commonly used technique. With deep hypothermic circulatory arrest, the patient is cooled to 18°C and circulation to the entire body is stopped during distal aortic reconstruction. This technique is safe and effective, but rather time consuming, and in some series, associated with higher blood product use. In a recent report by Ziganshin and colleagues,[51] the stroke rate of 490 patients undergoing aortic arch surgery was 1.6% (n = 8); however, those with deep hypothermic circulatory arrest times more than 50 minutes experienced a higher stroke rate. Retrograde cerebral perfusion involves fairly deep hypothermia while perfusing the cerebral circulation in a retrograde fashion through the venous circulation (superior vena cava to internal jugular vein). This technique has fallen out of favor at most centers. Antegrade cerebral perfusion has become the cerebral protection method of choice at most aortic centers. This technique involves moderate hypothermia (24–28°C) with cannulation of the axillary or innominate artery, which allows flow to be maintained to the brain during distal aortic reconstruction. Okita and colleagues[52] have shown this technique to reduce neurologic deficits. The authors prefer antegrade cerebral perfusion at their center.

After prompt transport to the operating room and induction of anesthesia, TEE is performed to confirm the diagnosis as well as assess the aortic valve and root. The authors cannulate the right axillary artery to facilitate cerebral perfusion during distal aortic reconstruction. After establishing cardiopulmonary bypass, cardiac arrest is induced, and the midportion of the ascending aorta is transected. They then inspect the proximal aorta to determine if root replacement or ascending aortic replacement is necessary. As long as the intimal tear does not extend below the sinotubular junction, simple supracoronary ascending aortic replacement is typically adequate. If there is a dissection flap remaining in the proximal aorta, it is obliterated with felt or similar material, and the proximal reconstruction with an appropriately sized vascular graft is completed (**Box 2**, **Figs. 5–11**). During this time, the authors continue to cool the patient for distal aortic reconstruction.

Once proximal reconstruction is completed and adequate cooling has been achieved, the innominate artery is clamped and antegrade cerebral perfusion is established. The goal is to perfuse the brain at a flow of about 10 mL/kg/min, which generally results in a cerebral perfusion pressure between 40 and 60 mm Hg. After initiation of circulatory arrest, the aortic cross-clamp is removed and the aortic arch is inspected for tears. The decision to proceed with hemiarch versus total arch is made based on the presence or absence of tear in the arch. The false lumen is again obliterated, and the distal anastomosis is completed (see also **Box 2**, **Figs. 5–10**; **Fig. 12**). The graft is then deaired; rewarming commences, and the patient is weaned from cardiopulmonary bypass. These patients are generally quite coagulopathic and require aggressive blood factor replacement to achieve adequate hemostasis.

POSTOPERATIVE AND LONG-TERM MANAGEMENT

Initial postoperative management focuses on hemodynamic management and assessment of end organ function. Most patients are hypertensive postoperatively and require aggressive antihypertensive management. Careful attention to renal and liver function is imperative, in addition to peripheral pulses and close observation of lower or upper extremity compartment syndrome, especially if there was limb malperfusion preoperatively. Patients are quickly weaned from sedation to assess neurologic function. Stroke remains a significant risk with aortic dissection repair and must be managed aggressively. In the uncomplicated patient, average hospital stay is 10 to 14 days. Any postoperative complications can of course extend this length of time significantly.

Long-term management is focused on the assessment of the remaining aorta. As most patients have a residual dissection flap in the aortic arch and/or descending aorta, serial CTA is required. The authors obtain a CTA on every patient 3 months postoperatively. If there is a

---

Box 2
Case report

A 56-year-old man with a history of hypertension presented to the emergency room with the acute onset of chest pain. He reported he had stopped taking his antihypertensive medications approximately 3 weeks prior because he ran out and could not afford to have them refilled. The patient was hemodynamically stable and neurologically intact; however, his blood pressure was 180/100. There were no other pertinent findings on physical examination. Chest pain evaluation revealed a normal ECG, normal chest radiograph, and normal cardiac enzymes. A CTA of the chest was obtained, which showed an acute type A aortic dissection (see **Fig. 5**). Note the 2 distinct lumens on CTA as well as evidence of 2 lumens in both the ascending and the descending aorta. The presence of the dissection flap in the ascending aorta confirms the diagnosis of a type A aortic dissection. The patient was taken to the operating room emergently. The aortic was visibly discolored consistent with an aortic dissection (see **Fig. 6**). An intimal tear was found in the midportion of the ascending aorta (see **Fig. 7**). The dissection flap ended proximally at the sinotubular junction, and the aortic valve was normal (see **Fig. 8**). Proximal reconstruction was completed, followed by distal reconstruction. For distal reconstruction, antegrade cerebral perfusion via the axillary artery was used for brain protection. The distal aorta was resected to the undersurface of the arch (so-called hemiarch); the false lumen was obliterated, and the graft was sewn in place (see **Fig. 9**). **Fig. 10** shows the completed reconstruction. The patient had an uneventful postoperative course.

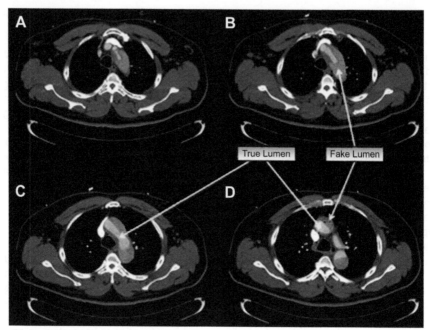

Fig. 5. CTA of acute type A aortic dissection. Sections (*A–C*) are at the aortic arch level, whereas section (*D*) is at the level of the pulmonary bifurcation. Note the separate 2 lumens in the aorta; in section (*D*), note the 2 lumen in both the ascending and the descending aorta. The presence of the dissection in the ascending aorta confirms the diagnosis of a type A aortic dissection.

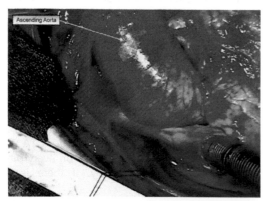

Fig. 6. Intraoperative image of ascending aorta. Note discoloration of ascending aorta, which is typical of an aortic dissection.

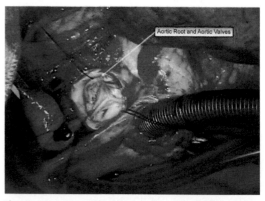

Fig. 8. Intraoperative image of proximal aorta. Note the dissection has ended above the aortic valve. Also note the normal-appearing aortic valve.

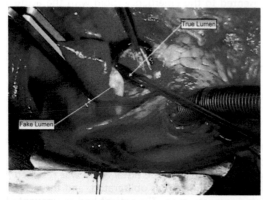

Fig. 7. Intraoperative image of opening ascending aorta. Note there are 2 distinct lumens in the ascending aorta. The lumen with blood clot present is the false lumen.

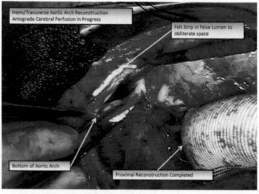

Fig. 9. Intraoperative image of distal aorta and undersurface of aortic arch. Note the false lumen, which is being obliterated with felt before reconstruction.

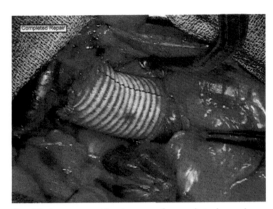

Fig. 10. Intraoperative image of completed repair.

residual dissection, they obtain repeat imaging at least every 6 months for the first 1 or 2 years. If the findings are stable, they will extend this to a yearly interval. If there are changes, they either consider intervention or increase the frequency of imaging to every 3 months. The management of the residual dissection after repair of a type A aortic dissection is beyond the scope of this article, but the reader is referred to the other articles in this issue.

CONTEMPORARY OUTCOMES

Although early reports of perioperative mortalities after repair of type A aortic dissection were 30% to 60%, contemporary results have improved, with most recent reports demonstrating a perioperative mortality of 13% to 25%.[1] In the most recent report from the International Registry of Acute Aortic Dissection, there was a 25% in-hospital mortality after repair of an acute type A aortic dissection. Long-term survival has been

reported to be in the range of 70% to 75% at 5 and 10 years in several studies. Kazui and colleagues[53] reported overall survival of 76% and 71% at 5 and 10 years, respectively, whereas Concistrè and colleagues[54] reported survival of 77%, 73%, and 62% at 1, 5, and 14 years. In the authors' recent experience of 196 patients undergoing repair of acute type A aortic dissection, in-hospital mortality was 9.7%. With a mean of 31 months follow-up, overall survival was 85.2%, 83.9%, 79.2%, and 74.7% at 6, 12, 36, and 60 months.

Predictors of mortality vary between studies, but the concept that shock, preoperative ischemia or malperfusion, advanced age, and previous cardiac surgery portend worse outcomes is worth emphasizing. In the International Registry of Acute Aortic Dissection report, those with a history of aortic valve replacement, migrating chest pain, shock, tamponade, and preoperative ischemia had worse outcomes.[55] In the authors' own series, the need for concomitant coronary artery bypass grafting, an intraoperative thoracic stent, and the development of postoperative renal failure requiring renal replacement therapy were risk factors for overall mortality.

The extent of proximal and distal aortic repair necessary for a durable repair in type A aortic dissection remains controversial. The authors found that neither the proximal nor the distal extent of the repair affects overall outcomes. Multiple other reports have shown similar survival with aortic root replacement and supracoronary aorta replacement,[56,57] which suggest that if aortic root replacement is required in the setting of acute type A aortic dissection, it is not associated with worse outcomes, and in some cases, may be preferable.[57]

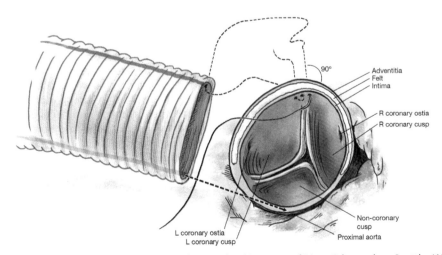

Fig. 11. Proximal reconstruction technique. L, left; R, right. (*Courtesy of* Mesa Schumacher, Seattle, WA.)

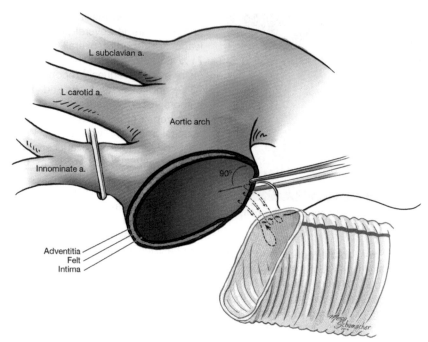

Fig. 12. Distal "hemiarch" reconstruction technique. a., artery. (*Courtesy of* Mesa Schumacher, Seattle, WA.)

Although the authors prefer to perform a hemiarch except in the setting of tear extending into the aortic arch or a branch vessel, others prefer a more aggressive "total arch" approach regardless of the location of the intimal tear. The optimal treatment of the distal aorta remains a matter of debate. The advantage of a "tear-directed approach" is in simplifying a complex emergent operation, while those that support a more aggressive approach think that aggressive arch replacement results in fewer long-term aortic interventions, at the expense of a more difficult operation in the emergent setting.

There are data to support both approaches. Several groups have shown equivalent survival rates between those undergoing hemiarch and total arch replacement at 5 years.[53] Kim and colleagues[58] found 5-year survival was superior in those with a hemiarch repair compared with the total arch replacement group (83.2 vs 65.8%) and that after inverse probability of treatment weighing, total arch patients were at greater risk of death and irreversible neurologic injury.

Preoperative malperfusion adds a dimension of complexity and increased mortality to repair of the acute type A aortic dissection. Augoustides and his group[59] developed a classification system of preoperative ischemia that groups patients into 4 groups: no ischemia, branch vessel malperfusion with localized organ ischemia, generalized ischemia with circulatory collapse, or a combination of both localized and generalized ischemia.[59] Using this classification system, Olsson and colleagues[60] reviewed 360 patients with acute type A aortic dissection and found localized or generalized ischemia to be independently associated with intraoperative and in-hospital mortality (see **Fig. 3**).

FUTURE DIRECTION

Technology has the potential to alter the manner in which acute type A aortic dissection is managed in the very near future. The technological advances and widespread adoption of endovascular repair of the aorta is now being extended to the proximal aorta and aortic arch. Nienaber and coworkers[61] recently published their early results of endovascular repair for acute type A aortic dissection using currently available stents in 12 poor surgical candidates and demonstrated technical success in 91% of patients. Although the technology needs to evolve further to better conform to the unique anatomic requirements of the aortic root, ascending aorta, and aortic arch, endoscopic therapy for acute type A aortic dissection is promising and has the potential to revolutionize its treatment.

SUMMARY

In summary, type A aortic dissection is a surgical emergency that requires prompt diagnosis and surgical treatment to optimize outcomes. Surgical repair requires replacement of the ascending aorta with or without aortic root and/or aortic arch replacement. Surgical outcomes for this highly lethal diagnosis have improved, with contemporary survival to discharge at Centers of Excellence of 85% to 90%. However, survival is highly related to prompt treatment, preexisting medical comorbidities, presence or absence of end organ malperfusion (kidney, brain, limb, abdominal), extent of aortic repair required, and the development of postoperative complications. Five-year survival rates of 70% to 80% after repair of type A aortic dissection are reported. Surgical results will need to be the benchmark for trials designed to evaluate the emerging field of endovascular repair for type A aortic dissection.

REFERENCES

1. Mussa FF, Horton JD, Moridzadeh R, et al. Acute aortic dissection and intramural hematoma. JAMA 2016;316(7):754–810.
2. Landenhed M, Engstrom G, Gottsater A, et al. Risk profiles for aortic dissection and ruptured or surgically treated aneurysms: a prospective cohort study. J Am Heart Assoc 2014;4(1):e001513.
3. Ewing MJ, Houck PD, Drake GB, et al. Mycotic pseudoaneurysm of the aortic arch with purulent pericardial effusion. Ann Thorac Surg 2012;93(4):1301–3.
4. Sullivan MKL, Steiner RM, Smullens SN, et al. Pseudoaneurysm of the ascending aorta following cardiac surgery. Chest 2015;93(1):138–43.
5. Debakey ME, Henly WS, Cooley DA, et al. Surgical management of dissecting aneurysms of the aorTA. J Thorac Cardiovasc Surg 1965;49:130–49.
6. DeBakey ME, McCollum CH, Crawford ES, et al. Dissection and dissecting aneurysms of the aorta: twenty-year follow-up of five hundred twenty-seven patients treated surgically. Surgery 1982;92(6):1118–34.
7. Coady MA, Rizzo JA, Goldstein LJ, et al. Natural history, pathogenesis, and etiology of thoracic aortic aneurysms and dissections. Cardiol Clin 1999;17(4):615–35, vii.
8. Manzur MF, Han SM, Dunn J, et al. Management of patients with acute aortic syndrome through a regional rapid transport system. J Vasc Surg 2017;65(1):21–9.
9. Aggarwal B, Raymond C, Jacob J, et al. Transfer of patients with suspected acute aortic syndrome. Am J Cardiol 2013;112(3):430–5.
10. Bickerstaff LK, Pairolero PC, Hollier LH, et al. Thoracic aortic aneurysms: a population-based study. Surgery 1982;92(6):1103–8.
11. Clouse WD, Hallett JW, Schaff HV, et al. Acute aortic dissection: population-based incidence compared with degenerative aortic aneurysm rupture. Mayo Clin Proc 2004;79:176–80.
12. Bossone E, Pyeritz RE, O'Gara P, et al. Acute aortic dissection in blacks: insights from the international registry of acute aortic dissection. Am J Med 2013;126(10):909–15.
13. Svensson LG, Labib SB, Eisenhauer AC, et al. Intimal tear without hematoma: an important variant of aortic dissection that can elude current imaging techniques. Circulation 1999;99(10):1331–6.
14. Larson EW, Edwards WD. Risk factors for aortic dissection: a necropsy study of 161 cases. Am J Cardiol 1984;53(6):849–55.
15. Harris KM, Braverman AC, Eagle KA, et al. Acute aortic intramural hematoma: an analysis from the International Registry of Acute Aortic Dissection. Circulation 2012;126(11 Suppl 1):S91–6.
16. Stanson AW, Kazmier FJ, Hollier LH, et al. Penetrating atherosclerotic ulcers of the thoracic aorta: natural history and clinicopathologic correlations. Ann Vasc Surg 1986;1(1):15–23.
17. Ganaha F, Miller DC, Sugimoto K, et al. Prognosis of aortic intramural hematoma with and without penetrating atherosclerotic ulcer: a clinical and radiological analysis. Circulation 2002;106(3):342–8.
18. Wada H, Sakata N, Tashiro T. Clinicopathological study on penetrating atherosclerotic ulcers and aortic dissection: distinct pattern of development of initial event. Heart Vessels 2016;31(11):1855–61.
19. Lansman SL, McCullough JN, Nguyen KH, et al. Subtypes of acute aortic dissection. Ann Thorac Surg 1999;67(6):1975–8 [discussion: 1979–80].
20. Coady MA, Rizzo JA, Elefteriades JA. Pathologic variants of thoracic aortic dissections: penetrating atherosclerotic ulcers and intramural hematomas. Cardiol Clin 1999;17(4):637–57.
21. Hirst AEJ, Johns VJJ, Kime SWJ. Dissecting aneurysm of the aorta: a review of 505 cases. Medicine (Baltimore) 1958;37(3):217–79.
22. Goldfinger JZ, Halperin JL, Marin ML, et al. Thoracic aortic aneurysm and dissection. J Am Coll Cardiol 2014;64(16):1725–39.
23. Mehta RH, O'Gara P, Bossone E, et al. Acute type A aortic dissection in the elderly: clinical characteristics, management, and outcomes in the current era. J Am Coll Cardiol 2002;40:1–9.
24. Hardean A, Biren M, Coralie S, et al. Ascending thoracic aneurysms are associated with decreased systemic atherosclerosis. Chest 2015;128(3):1580–6.
25. Hagan PG, Nienaber CA, Isselbacher EM, et al. The International Registry of Acute Aortic Dissection (IRAD): new insights into an old disease. JAMA 2000;283(7):897–903.
26. Yin H, Pickering GJ. Cellular senescence and vascular disease: novel routes to better understanding and therapy. Can J Cardiol 2016;32(5):612–23.

27. Kamel H, Roman MJ, Pitcher A, et al. Pregnancy and the risk of aortic dissection or rupture: a cohort-crossover analysis. Circulation 2016;134(7):527–33.

28. Sawlani N, Shroff A, Vidovich MI. Aortic dissection and mortality associated with pregnancy in the United States. J Am Coll Cardiol 2015;65(15):1600–1.

29. Ziganshin BA, Bailey AE, Coons C, et al. Routine genetic testing for thoracic aortic aneurysm and dissection in a clinical setting. Ann Thorac Surg 2015;100(5):1604–11.

30. Nienaber CA, Clough RE, Sakalihasan N, et al. Aortic dissection. Nat Publishing Group 2016;2:1–18.

31. Pepin M, Schwarze U, Superti-Fugra A, et al. Clinical and genetic features of Ehlers–Danlos syndrome type IV, the vascular type. N Engl J Med 2000;342(10):1–9.

32. Babatasi G, Massetti M, Bhoyroo S, et al. Pregnancy with aortic dissection in Ehler–Danlos syndrome. Staged replacement of the total aorta (10-year follow-up). Eur J Cardiothorac Surg 1997;12(4):671–4.

33. Gravholt CH, Landin-Wilhelmsen K, Stochholm K, et al. Clinical and epidemiological description of aortic dissection in Turner's syndrome. Cardiol Young 2006;16(05):430–8.

34. Lin AE, Lippe B, Rosenfield RG. Further delineation of aortic dilation, dissection, and rupture in patients with Turner syndrome. Pediatrics 1998;102:1–11.

35. Turtle EJ, Sule AA, Webb DJ, et al. Aortic dissection in children and adolescents with Turner syndrome: risk factors and management recommendations. Arch Dis Child 2015;100(7):662–6.

36. Mery CM, Reece T, Kron IL. Chapter 50. Aortic Dissection. In: Cohn LH, editor. Cardiac Surgery in the Adult. 4th edition. New York: McGraw-Hill; 2012. p. 1–39.

37. Núñez-Gil IJ, Bautista D, Cerrato E, et al. Incidence, Management, and Immediate- and Long-Term Outcomes After Iatrogenic Aortic Dissection During Diagnostic or Interventional Coronary Procedures. Circulation 2015;131(24):2114–9.

38. Nuenninghoff DM, Hunder GG, Christianson TJH, et al. Mortality of large-artery complication (aortic aneurysm, aortic dissection, and/or large-artery stenosis) in patients with giant cell arteritis: a population-based study over 50 years. Arthritis Rheum 2003;48(12):3532–7.

39. Wang SH, Chang YS, Liu CJ, et al. Incidence and risk analysis of aortic aneurysm and aortic dissection among patients with systemic lupus erythematosus: a nationwide population-based study in Taiwan. Lupus 2014;23(7):665–71.

40. Hiratzka LF, Bakris GL, Beckman JA, et al. 2010 ACCF/AHA/AATS/ACR/ASA/SCA/SCAI/SIR/STS/SVM guidelines for the diagnosis and management of patients with thoracic aortic disease. J Am Coll Cardiol 2010;55(14):e27–129.

41. Davies RR, Goldstein LJ, Coady MA, et al. Yearly rupture or dissection rates for thoracic aortic aneurysms: simple prediction based on size. Ann Thorac Surg 2002;73(1):17–27.

42. Chau KH, Elefteriades JA. Natural history of thoracic aortic aneurysms: size matters, plus moving beyond size. Prog Cardiovasc Dis 2013;56(1):74–80.

43. Demers P, Miller DC. Chapter 70-type A aortic dissection. 9th Edition. Philadelphia: Elsevier Inc.; 2016. p. 1214–43.

44. Pourafkari L, Tajlil A, Ghaffari S, et al. The frequency of initial misdiagnosis of acute aortic dissection in the emergency department and its impact on outcome. Intern Emerg Med 2016;1–11.

45. Hagan PG, Nienaber CA, Isselbacher EM, et al. The International Registry of Acute Aortic Dissection (IRAD): new insights into an old disease. JAMA 2000;283(7):897–903.

46. Czerny M, Schoenhoff F, Etz C, et al. The impact of pre-operative malperfusion on outcome in acute type A aortic dissection. J Am Coll Cardiol 2015;65(24):2628–35.

47. Hachulla A-L, Ronot M, Noble S, et al. ECG-triggered high-pitch CT for simultaneous assessment of the aorta and coronary arteries. J Cardiovasc Comput Tomogr 2016;10(5):407–13.

48. Evangelista A, Garcia-del-Castillo H, Gonzalez-Alujas T, et al. Diagnosis of ascending aortic dissection by transesophageal echocardiography: utility of M-mode in recognizing artifacts. J Am Coll Cardiol 1996;27(1):102–7.

49. Cecconi M, Chirillo F, Costantini C, et al. The role of transthoracic echocardiography in the diagnosis and management of acute type A aortic syndrome. Am Heart J 2012;163(1):112–8.

50. Cohen RG, Hackmann AE, Fleischman F, et al. Type A Aortic Dissection: How I Teach It. Ann Thorac Surg 2017;103(1):14–7.

51. Ziganshin BA, Rajbanshi BG, Tranquilli M, et al. Straight deep hypothermic circulatory arrest for cerebral protection during aortic arch surgery: safe and effective. J Thorac Cardiovasc Surg 2014;148(3):888–900.

52. Okita Y, Miyata H, Motomura N, et al, The Japan Cardiovascular Surgery Database Organization. A study of brain protection during total arch replacement comparing antegrade cerebral perfusion versus hypothermic circulatory arrest, with or without retrograde cerebral perfusion: analysis based on the Japan adult cardiovascular surgery database. J Thorac Cardiovasc Surg 2015;149(2 Suppl):S65–73.

53. Kazui T, Washiyama N, Bashar AHM, et al. Surgical outcome of acute type A aortic dissection: analysis of risk factors. Ann Thorac Surg 2002;74:75–82.

54. Concistrè G, Casali G, Santaniello E, et al. Reoperation after surgical correction of acute type A aortic dissection: risk factor analysis. Ann Thorac Surg 2012;93(2):450–5.

55. Trimarchi S, Nienaber CA, Rampoldi V, et al. Contemporary results of surgery in acute type A aortic dissection: the International Registry of Acute

Aortic Dissection experience. J Thorac Cardiovasc Surg 2005;129(1):112–22.

56. Halstead J, Spielvogel D, Meier D, et al. Composite aortic root replacement in acute type A dissection: time to rethink the indications? Eur J Cardiothorac Surg 2005;27(4):626–32.

57. Di Eusanio M, Trimarchi S, Peterson MD, et al. Root replacement surgery versus more conservative management during type A acute aortic dissection repair. Ann Thorac Surg 2014;98(6): 2078–84.

58. Kim JB, Chung CH, Moon DH, et al. Total arch repair versus hemiarch repair in the management of acute DeBakey type I aortic dissection. Eur J Cardiothorac Surg 2011;40(4):881–7.

59. Augoustides JG, Geirsson A, Szeto WY, et al. Observational study of mortality risk stratification by ischemic presentation in patients with acute type A aortic dissection: the Penn classification. Nat Clin Pract Cardiovasc Med 2008;6(2): 140–6.

60. Olsson C, Hillebrant CG, Liska J, et al. Mortality in acute type A aortic dissection: validation of the penn classification. Ann Thorac Surg 2011;92(4): 1376–82.

61. Nienaber CA, Sakalihasan N, Clough RE, et al. Thoracic endovascular aortic repair (TEVAR) in proximal (type A) aortic dissection: ready for a broader application? J Thorac Cardiovasc Surg 2017;153(2):S3–11.

Diagnostic and Treatment Dilemmas of the Aortic Arch

 CrossMark

Dawn S. Hui, MD[a],*, Fernando Fleischman, MD[b]

KEYWORDS

- Aortic arch • Aortic aneurysm • Endovascular • Thoracic stent graft

KEY POINTS

- The aortic arch remains the last frontier for endovascular treatment, with unique anatomic and hemodynamic features posing special challenges to safe, durable repairs.
- Although total endovascular options for treatment of aortic arch abnormality are on the horizon of commercial availability, outcomes are subject to heterogeneity of studies and limited data.
- High-volume centers with aortic expertise continue to report improving outcomes for open aortic arch repair, the standard against which hybrid repair should be judged in both the short and the long term.

INTRODUCTION

The history of surgical repair of aortic arch aneurysms has been marked by improvements in anesthetic, surgical, and neuroprotective techniques. However, it remains an operation with the potential for significant morbidity and mortality, due to the physiologic and neurologic effects associated with cardiopulmonary bypass (CPB) and deep hypothermic circulatory arrest (DHCA). In addition, patients with aortic arch abnormalities often have features that increase surgical risk, such as advanced age, systemic comorbidities, or prior sternotomy, particularly with arch aneurysms after repair of an acute aortic dissection. Although case reports of surgical aortic arch repair without DHCA and CPB have been presented,[1–3] endovascular approaches are appealing for their minimally invasive nature, in addition to minimization or avoidance of CPB and DHCA.

The goals of endovascular repair of arch aneurysms are to completely exclude the aneurysm sac, avoid atheroemboli, and preserve perfusion of the supra-aortic branches. Unique anatomic and hemodynamic features of the arch pose special challenges to achieving these goals (**Table 1**).

Curvature and Angulation

An underlying principle for durability of endovascular stent grafting is the presence of a seal zone that has healthy aorta free of calcification and thrombus, parallel walls or minimal tapering, angulation less than 60°, and adequate length. Without these optimal conditions, proximal seal and stent conformity are imperfect and subject to compromise of long-term integrity. Furthermore, the dynamic strain of the arch curvature can lead to stent complications, such as migration, kinking, or fracture. Ishimaru zones 1 and 2 rarely meet the conditions for an ideal landing zone, necessitating a strategy for either extra-anatomic bypass, or fenestrated or multibranched graft procedures.

The authors have no financial interests to disclose.
[a] Department of Surgery, Center for Comprehensive Cardiovascular Care, Saint Louis University, 3635 Vista Avenue, DT 13th Floor, St Louis, MO 63130, USA; [b] Department of Cardiothoracic Surgery, Keck School of Medicine, University of Southern California, 1520 San Pablo Street, HCC II, Suite 4300, Los Angeles, CA 90033, USA
* Corresponding author.
E-mail address: huids@slu.edu

Table 1
Unique characteristics of the aortic arch

Factor	Endovascular Concerns
Arch curvature	Trackability and conformity
	Endograft apposition, seal
Greater pulsatility and flow, dynamic strain	Risk of stent migration, kinking, or fracture
	Windsock movement of endograft before fixation
Supra-aortic branching	Cerebrovascular perfusion
	Landing zone limitations
Procedural	Atheroemboli, vascular injury, retrograde type A dissection

Hemodynamic Load

Compared with the descending thoracic and abdominal portions of the aorta, the aortic arch has greater pulsatility and higher blood flow.

Pulsatile strain can occur in both the longitudinal and the circumferential directions but is theorized to be greater in the longitudinal direction, explaining the aortic elongation seen with aging.[4] The supra-aortic branches have relatively lower pulsatility, due to tethering to other anatomic structures. These hemodynamic factors have implications for long-term stent performance, including disconnection of modular devices.

Supra-aortic Branching

In addition to the challenges posed by arch curvature, the proximity of the branch vessel ostia is a major factor in evaluating Ishimaru zones 1 and 2 as adequate landing zones (**Fig. 1**A). The catastrophic consequences of covering the origin of a supra-aortic branch mandate precision in alignment and deployment. Bergeron and colleagues[5] have proposed an alternate classification scheme of landing zones relative to these ostia (**Fig. 1**B). Throughout the remainder of the discussion, the Ishimaru classification will be used.

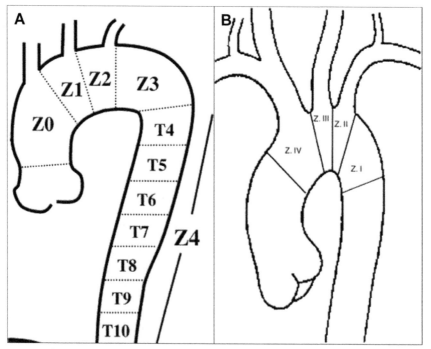

Fig. 1. (*A*) Anatomy of the aortic arch with Ishimaru classification of landing zones. Zone 0, ascending aorta up to the brachiocephalic artery; zone 1, between the brachiocephalic artery and LCCA; zone 2, between the LCCA and LSCA; zone 3, proximal descending thoracic aorta distal to LSCA; zone 4, middescending thoracic aorta. (*B*) Retrograde landing zone classification proposed by Bergeron, with zone 1 distal to LSCA; zone 2 lies between the LSCA and LCCA; zone 3 between the LCCA and innominate artery; zone 4 is the ascending aorta up to the brachiocephalic artery. (*From* Moon MC, Morales JP, Greenberg RK. The aortic arch and ascending aorta: are they within the endovascular realm? Semin Vasc Surg 2007;20(2):103; and Bergeron P, Mangialardi N, Costa P, et al. Great vessel management for endovascular exclusion of aortic arch aneurysms and dissections. Eur J Vasc Endovasc Surg 2006;32(1):41, with permission.)

Procedural and Technical Factors

Minimally invasive approaches do not necessarily translate to minimal risk outcomes. In addition to the well-known risks of endovascular procedures such as contrast-induced nephropathy, radiation exposure, and vascular injury, endovascular procedures to treat the aortic arch pose unique risks of neurologic injury. Atheroma residing in the arch and supra-aortic branches, as well as aortic valve calcification, may give rise to emboli from the interaction of wires, devices, and delivery systems. With transfemoral access, a longer distance to the target area is a limitation to precise control of the proximal device end. Auto-aligning features of branched and fenestrated stent grafts help reduce the manipulation needed for accurate positioning. Finally, spinal cord ischemia is a risk, depending on the extent of coverage of the descending thoracic aorta.

Despite these daunting challenges, technological developments have progressed such that total endovascular options are in the realm of feasibility. This evolution has developed through greater incorporation of and experience with endovascular technology; advancements in design and procedural technique have increased the safety and long-term outcome profiles. However, a more "minimally invasive" approach still carries specific procedural risks, as outlined above, and long-term outcome data are extremely limited at this time. Furthermore, the individualized approach generally required for such complex patients means that comparative data of various techniques, to say nothing of randomized trials, will be slow to accumulate. Finally, one should bear in mind that with continued improvements in open aortic arch surgery, contemporary outcomes are excellent[6–8] with 30-day mortality of 5% to 9.7% and stroke incidence of 2.8% to 6.2%. These contemporary outcomes of open aortic surgery are the standards against which hybrid and endovascular approaches should be compared.

Surgical techniques

At present, total endovascular treatment of the aortic arch is in its nascency, with commercial devices not yet available in the United States. The primary role of endovascular technology is as part of a hybrid approach combined with open surgical techniques (**Fig. 2**). Here, a brief review of the terminology may be useful (**Fig. 3**).

Hybrid arch type I repair

For aneurysms isolated to the arch with healthy zones 0 and 3/4 appropriate for landing, extra-anatomic inflow to the supra-aortic branches is

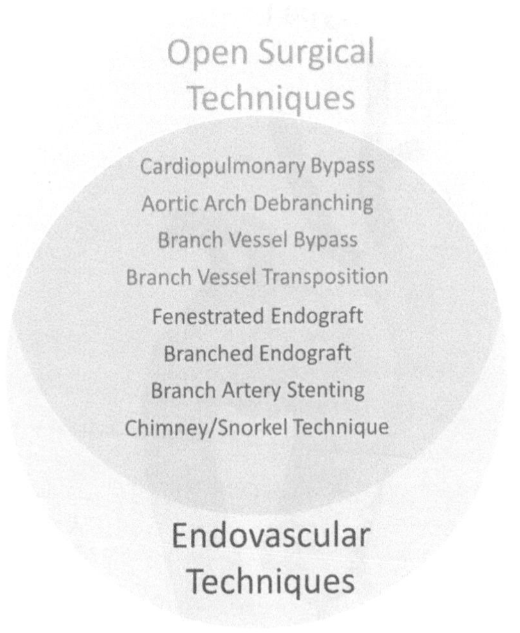

Open Surgical Techniques

Cardiopulmonary Bypass
Aortic Arch Debranching
Branch Vessel Bypass
Branch Vessel Transposition
Fenestrated Endograft
Branched Endograft
Branch Artery Stenting
Chimney/Snorkel Technique

Endovascular Techniques

Fig. 2. Open surgical and endovascular techniques used in hybrid treatment of aortic arch disease.

established in native proximal ascending aorta. This branch inflow revascularization can be performed with a single branched graft. Other variations of inflow to the various branches are outlined in later discussion (see Management of supra-aortic branches).

Hybrid arch type II repair

When aneurysmal disease involves the aorta proximal to the innominate artery, achieving a good seal and sizing of the graft are of concern; furthermore, there is a significant risk of retrograde type A dissection. Accordingly, the proximal ascending aorta is replaced to when the ascending aorta is aneurysmal (with a threshold as low as 3.7 cm in some institutions).[9] This operation generally requires CPB and possibly DHCA with cerebral perfusion.

Hybrid arch type III repair

The usual indication for type III repairs is mega-aortic syndrome, with diffuse aneurysmal disease of the ascending aorta, aortic arch, and descending thoracic aorta. Open replacement of the ascending aorta and transverse arch with an elephant trunk comprise stage I, followed by retrograde endovascular deployment of a stent graft into the elephant trunk.

Management of supra-aortic branches

Extra-anatomic bypass, initially proposed to treat occlusive disease of the innominate or carotid

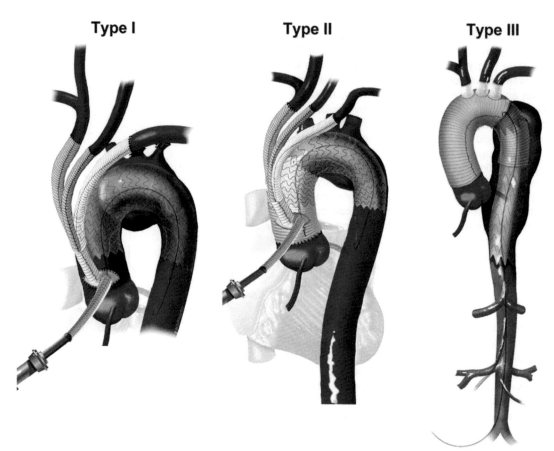

Type I　　**Type II**　　**Type III**

Fig. 3. Hybrid arch repair types. (*From* Bavaria J, Vallabhajosyula P, Moeller P, et al. Hybrid approaches in the treatment of aortic arch aneurysms: postoperative and midterm outcomes. J Thorac Cardiovasc Surg 2013;145(30):S87; with permission.)

vessels, has been used to extend the proximal landing zone of aortic endografts. Management of the left subclavian artery (LSCA) and left common carotid artery (LCCA) can be performed without sternotomy through cervical incisions alone.[5] Left subclavian revascularization by carotid-subclavian bypass affords landing in zone 2; carotid-carotid bypass extends the possibility of proximal coverage to zone 1 (**Fig. 4**). Sequential transpositions involving an upper hemi-sternotomy have also been described.[10] As a side note, these techniques are reliant on supra-aortic branches for inflow and are vulnerable to compromise should occlusive disease progress. Although routine versus selective revascularization of the LSCA remains a topic of debate,[11,12] the current Society for Vascular Surgery guidelines recommend routine revascularization of the LSCA in elective cases and an individualized approach in urgent cases.[13] Preoperative imaging of the cerebral vasculature, including the circle of Willis, should be performed in all elective cases, with transposition or bypass procedures mandatory

for an existing left internal mammary graft, a stenotic or absent right vertebral artery, stenotic disease of the carotid arteries, or an incomplete circle of Willis. One advantage of not bypassing the LSCA is that it can serve as an access point to treat type I endoleaks. However, risks include left arm claudication or ischemia requiring revascularization, type II endoleaks from the LSCA, and posterior circulation strokes. In a large series, the rate of type II endoleaks arising from the LSCA was 7.5%.[14] The investigators also pointed out that posterior strokes, which in their series were comparable between LSCA coverage and revascularization (4.6% vs 3.6%), cannot be predicted even when normal intracerebral circulation is seen on preoperative imaging.

Management of zone 0

Given the anatomic constraints of the arch as a landing zone and the ensuing risk of endoleaks, one solution is to extend the proximal landing to zone 0, rerouting the supra-aortic branches by surgical transposition or bypass. This approach may

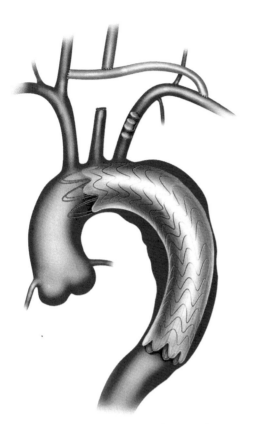

also be used when aortic arch disease requires coverage of the innominate artery, or the innominate artery has poor inflow to supply the LCCA. When the ascending aorta is free of disease (atheromatous plaque, calcification), total arch revascularization is performed via median sternotomy without CPB. A side-biting clamp is applied to the aorta for creation of the proximal anastomosis. A common approach is a trifurcated graft with separate distal anastomoses to each of the supra-aortic branches (see **Fig. 3**). A great number of variations have been reported, such as use of an inverse bifurcated graft anastomosed to the innominate and LCCA, followed by LCCA-LSCA transposition (**Fig. 5**),[15,16] or sequential transpositions (LSCA-LCCA, LCCA-right common carotid artery [RCCA]).[17,18] Ligation or coiling of the supraaortic stumps after a bypass procedure is mandatory to prevent endoleaks.[19] Supra-aortic rerouting without aortic manipulation has also been reported, with right axillary to left axillary and LCCA bypass.[20] Choice of technique should take into consideration risks of intrathoracic graft kinking due to retrosternal bulk, dependence on a single inflow limb to multiple branches versus inflow from supra-aortic branches, which may have occlusive disease, and patient tolerance for a sternotomy. When the ascending aorta is aneurysmal and if the patient can tolerate CPB, replacement of the ascending aorta is performed concomitantly to prevent retrograde dissection and proximal endoleaks. An additional step of a

Fig. 4. Carotid-carotid bypass, with extension to revascularize the LSCA. In addition, the LSCA has been occluded proximally. (*From* Andersen ND, Williams JB, Hanna JM, et al. Results with an algorithmic approach to hybrid repair of the aortic arch. J Vasc Surg 2013;57(3):657; with permission.)

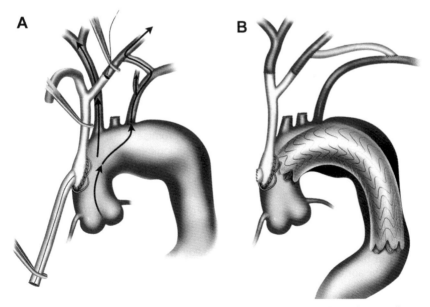

Fig. 5. Native zone 0 hybrid arch repair. (*A*) Initial construction of a left carotid-subclavian bypass allows uninterrupted left cerebral blood flow during left common carotid artery debranching. (*B*) Antegrade endovascular deployment occurs via the limb seen in panel A; this limb is subsequently oversewn. (*From* Andersen ND, Williams JB, Hanna JM, et al. Results with an algorithmic approach to hybrid repair of the aortic arch. J Vasc Surg 2013;57(3):658; with permission.)

limited ascending aortoplasty of the distal ascending aorta, in the region of the intended proximal deployment zone, has been used. Radiopaque markers placed during this procedure guide the second stage (**Fig. 6**). Aortoplasty can also be used as an alternative to graft replacement for aneurysmal ascending aortas when the patient is deemed too high risk for CPB.[15]

Reported contemporary outcomes for hybrid procedures combining arch debranching and endovascular stenting is shown in **Table 2**. Mortalities range from 6% to 11%, with a notably higher rate (27%) in a series that included 34% emergency cases.[24] There is a variation in practices such as the proportion of antegrade versus retrograde stenting, left subclavian revascularization, and the proportion and interval period of a metachronous strategy. In a multivariable analysis of 319 patients undergoing total arch replacement, Preventza and colleagues[25] reported no differences in operative mortality (10.3% overall),

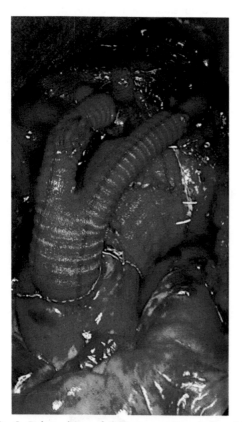

Fig. 6. Debranching of the supra-aortic vessels, with the reinforcement of the aorta of the supposed landing zone and radiopaque markers. (*From* Gelpi G, Vanelli P, Mangini A, et al. Hybrid aortic arch repair procedure: reinforcement of the aorta for a safe and durable landing zone. Eur J Vasc Endovasc Surg 2010;40(6):709–14; with permission.)

permanent stroke (5.9%), or long-term survival (78.7% at 4.5 years) in a propensity-matched comparison of open versus a hybrid zone 0 approach (25 pairs). In another propensity-matched study of 182 patients (38 propensity-matched pairs), Tokuda and colleagues[26] also demonstrated equivalent short-term results, although reporting operative, and not 30-day, mortality at 2.6% with hybrid versus 0% with open surgery. At follow-up, open repair had superior rates of freedom from aortic events (99% vs 79% at 24 months, $P<.0001$). The study did include type III hybrid arch repairs, in contrast to Preventza and colleagues, who only studied type I and type II repairs, again demonstrating the heterogeneity across studies. In both studies, 20 patients were not able to be matched, demonstrating that a substantial proportion of hybrid repair patients have no comparable open repair counterpart and highlighting the risk profile of these patients. On the other hand, Murashita and colleagues[27] found that of 191 open repair patients, 88 were not feasible to have a hybrid repair. As in the other studies, midterm survival at 2 years was not different between the 2 approaches.

Total endovascular approach

With advances in the design of endovascular systems for abdominal aorta disease, endograft stenting was initially extended to treat aneurysms of the descending thoracic aorta. Use of fenestrated stent grafts, branched stent grafts, and branch artery stents offer the possibility for a total endovascular option to treat the aortic arch (see Akiko Tanaka and Anthony Estrera's article, "Endovascular Treatment Options for the Aortic Arch," in this issue).

Future directions

Along with improvements in hybrid technology and outcomes and the approaching feasibility of total endovascular options, developments in imaging hold promise for a greater understanding of the physiologic impact of these treatment modalities. Two such examples are 4-dimensional flow MRI and computational fluid dynamics (CFD). One novel device that has received Conformité Européene mark is the Streamliner Multilayer Flow Modulator device (Cardiatis; Isnes, Brussels, Belgium), a braided mesh of highly flexible cobalt alloy wires that are high in resistance to kinking and fatigue, low in total porosity, and interconnected in multiple layers. Rather than complete exclusion of the aneurysm sac, the underlying principle of this platform is the modulation of turbulent laminar flow. The mesh configuration allows collateral branch patency. CFD was used to study

Table 2
Selected contemporary series of hybrid arch repairs

Author, Study Period	n	30-d or Inhospital Mortality (%)	Stroke (%)	Paraplegia (%)	Retrograde Type A Dissection	Reintervention (%)	Reported Survival, Follow-Up
Preventza et al,[15] 2005–2011	29	6.9	10.3	6.9	0	6.9	79.3% at 411 d
Ferrero et al,[17] 2005–2010	27	11.1	0	0	0	0	77.8% at 16.7 mo
Vallabhajosyula et al,[19] 2005–2012	47	8	8	5.5	2.7	2.7	71% at 1 y 60% at 3 y 48% at 5 y
Czerny et al,[21] 2003–2011	66	9	5	3	3	14	81% at 1 y 72% at 5 y
Hughes et al,[22] 2005–2008	28	0	0	3.6	0	7	70% at 3 y
Bavaria et al,[23] 2005–2009	27	11	11	7	—	0	
Geisbusch et al,[24] 1997–2009	47	19	6.3	6	6.3	27.6	77% at 1 y 59% at 3 y

clinical outcomes as well as simulate performance under different conditions.[28]

SUMMARY

Endovascular approaches to the aortic arch are challenged by unique anatomy and physiology of this area. Simple application of conventional endovascular technology and technique for abdominal or descending thoracic aortic disease to the aortic arch is insufficient to achieve effective and durable repairs. Appreciation of these challenges has led to developments in endovascular technology as well as complex strategies to deal with individual patient anatomy, that hold the potential for continued improved outcomes in both the short and the long term.

REFERENCES

1. Ishida N, Takemura H, Shimabukuro K, et al. Normothermic total arch replacement without hypothermic circulatory arrest to treat aortic distal arch aneurysm in a patient with cold agglutinin disease. Interact Cardiovasc Thorac Surg 2011;13:432–4.
2. Matalanis G, Koirala RS, Shi WY, et al. Branch first aortic arch replacement with no circulatory arrest or deep hypothermia. J Thorac Cardiovasc Surg 2011;142:809–15.
3. Marenchino RG, Domenech A. Single stage aortic arch replacement without circulatory arrest. Aorta (Stamford) 2016;4:29–31.
4. O'Rourke M, Farnsworth A, O'Rourke J. Aortic dimensions and stiffness in normal adults. JACC Cardiovasc Imaging 2008;1:749–51.
5. Bergeron P, Mangialardi N, Costa P, et al. Great vessel management for endovascular exclusion of aortic arch aneurysms and dissections. Eur J Vasc Endovasc Surg 2006;32:38–45.
6. Leshnower BG, Kilgo PD, Chen EP. Total arch replacement using moderate hypothermic circulatory arrest and unilateral selective antegrade cerebral perfusion. J Thorac Cardiovasc Surg 2014; 147:1488–92.
7. Patel HJ, Nguyen C, Diener AC, et al. Open arch reconstruction in the endovascular era: analysis of 721 patients over 17 years. J Thorac Cardiovasc Surg 2011;141:1417–23.
8. Thomas M, Li Z, Cook DJ, et al. Contemporary outcomes of open aortic arch surgery. J Thorac Cardiovasc Surg 2012;144:838–44.
9. Bavaria J, Vallabhajosyula P, Moeller P, et al. Hybrid approaches in the treatment of aortic arch aneurysms: postoperative and midterm outcomes. J Thorac Cardiovasc Surg 2013;145:S85–90.
10. Czerny M, Fleck T, Zimpfer D, et al. Combined repair of an aortic arch aneurysm by sequential transposition of the supra-aortic branches and endovascular stent-graft placement. J Thorac Cardiovasc Surg 2003;126:916–8.
11. Hajibandeh S, Hajibandeh S, Antoniou SA, et al. Revascularisation of the left subclavian artery for thoracic endovascular aortic repair. Cochrane Database Syst Rev 2016;(4):CD011738.
12. Dunning J, Martin JE, Shennib H, et al. Is it safe to cover the left subclavian artery when placing an endovascular stent in the descending thoracic aorta? Interact Cardiovasc Thorac Surg 2008;7:690–7.
13. Matsumura JS, Lee WA, Mitchell RS, et al. The Society for Vascular Surgery Practice Guidelines: management of the left subclavian artery with thoracic endovascular aortic repair. J Vasc Surg 2009;50: 1155–8.
14. Peterson MD, Wheatley GH 3rd, Kpodonu J, et al. Treatment of type II endoleaks associated with left subclavian artery coverage during thoracic aortic stent grafting. J Thorac Cardiovasc Surg 2008; 136(5):1193–9.
15. Preventza O, Aftab M, Coselli JS. Hybrid techniques for complex aortic arch surgery. Tex Heart Inst J 2013;40:568–71.
16. Preventza O, Bakaeen FG, Cervera RD, et al. Deployment of proximal thoracic endograft in zone 0 of the ascending aorta: treatment options and early outcomes for aortic arch aneurysms in a high-risk population. Eur J Cardiothorac Surg 2013;44:446–53.
17. Ferrero E, Ferri M, Viazzo A, et al. Is total debranching a safe procedure for extensive aortic-arch disease? A single experience of 27 cases. Eur J Cardiothorac Surg 2012;41:177–82.
18. Bergeron P, Coulon P, De Chaumaray T, et al. Great vessels transposition and aortic arch exclusion. J Cardiovasc Surg 2005;46:141–7.
19. Vallabhajosyula P, Szeto W, Desai N, et al. Type I and type II hybrid aortic arch replacement: postoperative and mid-term outcome analysis. Ann Cardiothorac Surg 2013;2:280–7.
20. Ryomoto M, Tanaka H, Kajiyama T, et al. Endovascular aortic arch repair with mini-cardiopulmonary bypass to prevent stroke. Ann Vasc Surg 2016;36: 320–4.
21. Czerny M, Weigang E, Sodeck G, et al. Targeting landing zone 0 by total arch rerouting and TEVAR: midterm results of a transcontinental registry. Ann Thorac Surg 2012;94:84–9.
22. Hughes GC, Daneshmand MA, Balsara KR, et al. "Hybrid" repair of aneurysms of the transverse aortic arch: midterm results. Ann Thorac Surg 2009;88: 1822–7.
23. Bavaria JE, Milewski RK, Baker J, et al. Classic hybrid evolving approach to distal arch aneurysms: toward the zone zero solution. J Thorac Cardiovasc Surg 2010;140:S77–80.

24. Geisbusch P, Kotelis D, Muller-Eschner M, et al. Complications after aortic arch hybrid repair. J Vasc Surg 2011;53:935–41.

25. Preventza O, Gracia A, Cooley DA, et al. Total aortic arch replacement: a comparative study of zone 0 hybrid arch exclusion versus traditional open repair. J Thorac Cardiovasc Surg 2015;150: 1591–600.

26. Tokuda Y, Oshima H, Narita Y, et al. Hybrid versus open repair of aortic arch aneurysms: comparison of postoperative and mid-term outcomes with a propensity score-matching analysis. Eur J Cardiothorac Surg 2016;49:149–56.

27. Murashita T, Matsuda H, Domae K, et al. Less invasive surgical treatment for aortic arch aneurysms in high-risk patients: a comparative study of hybrid thoracic endovascular aortic repair and conventional total arch replacement. J Thorac Cardiovasc Surg 2012;143:1007–13.

28. Stefanov F, Morris L, Elhelali A, et al. Insights from complex aortic surgery with a Streamliner device for aortic arch repair (STAR). J Thorac Cardiovasc Surg 2016;152:1309–18.

Endovascular Treatment Options for the Aortic Arch

Akiko Tanaka, MD, PhD, Anthony Estrera, MD*

KEYWORDS

- Aortic arch • Thoracic endovascular aortic repair • Hybrid procedure approach

KEY POINTS

- Endovascular aortic repair to treat aortic arch abnormality has rapidly expanded in the last 2 decades, and surgeons now have options to treat patients who are poor candidates for open surgery.
- The devices and techniques should be tailored to the extension of the aortic abnormality and anatomy of the individuals.
- Recent studies demonstrate promising results with branched endografts, but one of the major drawbacks of the devices is that considerable time is required to prepare the custom-made graft, which may not be available for emergent or urgent cases.
- Introduction of commercially available devices is forthcoming. In addition, the risk of stroke following endovascular repair of the aortic arch remains as high as for conventional open surgery.
- Until the long-term outcomes become available, the indications of endovascular treatment should be carefully considered in patients with low risk for open surgical repair, especially in young patients with connective tissue disorders.

INTRODUCTION

Thoracic endovascular aortic repair (TEVAR) has emerged as a less invasive alternative to conventional open surgery. Endografting techniques require a minimum 15-mm landing (sealing) zone proximally and distally and a minimum of 20 mm in a highly angulated arch to seal out the diseased aorta from the inside.[1] TEVAR for descending thoracic aortic aneurysms, in lesions with minimal anatomic restrictions, rapidly became the first-line treatment. At the same time, aneurysms of the aortic arch have been the "Achilles heel" of TEVAR[2] due to the vital branches to the brain, curvature of the arch, and high blood flow in the area.[3] Thanks to substantial advances in endovascular techniques and graft materials, there now are several options for endovascular aortic arch repair.

In this article, the authors discuss the current available endovascular repair techniques for the aortic arch abnormality.

Difficulties in Managing Aortic Arch Disease with Conventional Open Repair

Conventional open aortic arch repair requires a long cardiopulmonary bypass and circulatory arrest with deep hypothermia, which leads to inflammatory and ischemic insults to the patient. Contemporary studies have demonstrated that postoperative adverse events following open total arch replacement remain high: stroke was observed in 2.8% to 3.4%; prolonged ventilation (>48 hours) in 6% to 13.4%; and in-hospital mortality in 4.5% to 9.7%.[4–7] These results are reported from the experienced large-volume

Department of Cardiothoracic and Vascular Surgery, McGovern Medical School at The University of Texas Health Science Center at Houston (UTHealth) and Memorial Hermann Hospital, 6400 Fannin Street, Suite #2850, Houston, TX 77030, USA
* Corresponding author.
E-mail address: Anthony.L.Estrera@uth.tmc.edu

Cardiol Clin 35 (2017) 357–366
http://dx.doi.org/10.1016/j.ccl.2017.03.005
0733-8651/17/© 2017 Elsevier Inc. All rights reserved.

centers, and outcomes in the low-volume centers may even be worse. Thus, less invasive treatment options have been sought for the aortic arch abnormality, and innovative endovascular techniques have been used to conquer the anatomic challenges of the aortic arch.

HYBRID PROCEDURE APPROACH
Open Aortic Arch Repair with "Frozen Elephant Trunk"

There are 2 types of "hybrid" aortic arch repair. One type is open aortic arch repair with distal extension using the stent graft. This method is often referred to as "frozen elephant trunk,"[8] "stented elephant trunk,"[9] or "antegrade thoracic stent grafting."[10] Elephant trunk is the technique first reported by Borst and colleagues[11] in 1983 to treat extensive aortic aneurysm, in which a free "tangling" graft was left in the descending aortic aneurysm for the ease of the second-stage procedure. In 1996, Kato and colleagues[12] reported a successful experience with combined open surgical and endovascular aortic repair of the distal arch abnormality, modifying the classical elephant trunk technique. In their series, the stent graft was deployed as a replacement of conventional distal anastomosis of the aortic arch graft to reduce the pump and circulatory arrest time. This technique also enabled treatment of patients with extensive aortic aneurysm, involving the transverse arch and the descending aorta, with open aortic arch repair with antegrade stent grafting (**Fig. 1**). Although the original technique obviated a distal anastomosis, most of the current techniques prefer hand-sewing of the proximal end of the frozen elephant trunk (or the cuff) to avoid migration. To date, the frozen elephant trunk technique is indicated for extensive aortic aneurysms involving the transverse arch and descending aorta. It is also used to treat acute

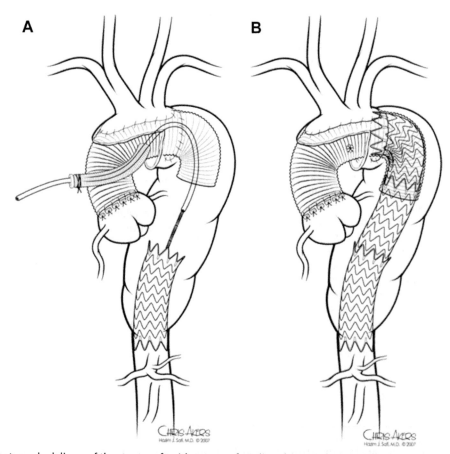

Fig. 1. Antegrade delivery of the stent graft without use of cardiopulmonary bypass. (*A*) Graft replacement of the ascending and transverse arch was completed using the elephant trunk technique. A stent graft is being deployed to the distal descending aorta through the side branch of the open repair graft. (*B*) Additional stent grafts were delivered to complete the aneurysm repair. (*Courtesy of* Chris Akers, MA, Memorial Hermann Hospital; Hazim J. Safi, MD, McGovern Medical School at UTHealth, Houston, TX.)

type A aortic dissection to reduce aneurysmal growth in the distal aorta.[13–15] Currently, there are 4 prefabricated hybrid prostheses available in the market outside the United States. The E-Vita Open and E-Vita Open Plus (JOTEC GmbH, Hechingen, Germany) have the longest history. Its international registry data from 2005 to 2014 (N = 509)[16] demonstrated in-hospital mortality of 16% for aortic dissection patients (81 of 350) and 13% for nondissection patients (21 of 159). They also reported postoperative stroke in 8% (41 of 509) and spinal cord injury in 8% (38 of 509; which was permanent in 4% [19 of 509]) with perioperative spinal fluid drainage used in 22% of the study. A distal landing zone lower than T10 was identified as an independent predictor of spinal cord injury (odds ratio [OR]: 2.3, 95% confidence interval [CI]: 1.1–4.9, P = .03). Recently, short-term outcomes of a 4-branched frozen elephant trunk hybrid prosthesis, Thoraflex (Vascutek, Inchinnan, United Kingdom),[17] was reported by a German group, which demonstrated similar results: 7% perioperative mortality; 7% spinal cord injury (1% permanent), with 100% use of perioperative spinal fluid drainage.

In early 2016, the clinical trial of Thoraflex Hybrid Device (Terumo Cardiovascular Group, Ann Arbor, MI, USA) was announced in the United States. The outcomes of E-Vita Open and Thoraflex suggest that frozen elephant trunk technique is a feasible option to treat a patient with transverse to proximal descending aortic aneurysm as a 1-stage procedure, but staged repair appears to have lower rates of spinal cord ischemia in patients with extensive aortic aneurysms.

Extra-Anatomic Bypass Combined with Thoracic Endografting

The other type of hybrid procedure is an extra-anatomic bypass involving the supra-aortic vessels combined with stent grafting to allow proximal extension of the landing zone. This technique is referred to as surgical "debranching" of the arch vessels. In the late 1990s, hybrid aortic arch repair without the use of cardiopulmonary bypass was reported.[18,19] These early studies used bypass from the ascending aorta to supra-aortic branches via median sternotomy. In 2000, an extrathoracic approach with left carotid to left subclavian artery bypass combined with TEVAR was reported for entry closure of acute type B aortic dissection.[20]

A treatment approach with hybrid debranching TEVAR is better understood with Ishimaru's anatomic classification of landing zones.[21,22] Zone 0 involves the ascending aorta and the innominate

artery origin; zone 1 involves the left common carotid artery origin; zone 2 involves the subclavian artery origin (**Fig. 2**). Debranching procedures can be performed with or without sternotomy with special consideration for zone 0 cases.

Zone 0 deployment is used when the aortic disease extends to the ascending aorta or proximal arch.[23] One option is a bypass from the ascending aorta to the innominate and left common carotid artery (**Fig. 3**). If the left subclavian artery is difficult to approach, it may be revascularized later with subclavian transposition or left subclavian-carotid artery bypass (**Fig. 4**). The endovascular repair is often performed as a concomitant procedure to extra-anatomic bypass because it allows antegrade deployment of the graft with more precise control.[24,25] The stent can be deployed in antegrade fashion through a branch of the bypass graft or retrograde via the femoral artery. When the size of the ascending aorta exceeds 3.7 cm, the ascending aorta is recommended to be

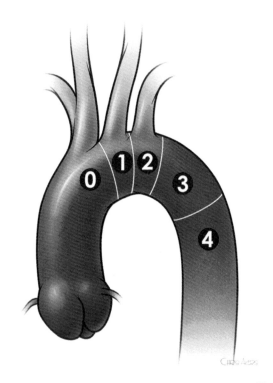

Fig. 2. Aortic arch zones established by Ishimaru.[21] Zone 0 involves the ascending aorta and the innominate artery origin; zone 1 involves the left common carotid artery origin; zone 2 involves the subclavian artery origin. The Society of Vascular Surgery defined the borderline of zone 3 and 4 as 2 cm distal to the subclavian artery origin.[22] (*Courtesy of* Chris Akers, MA, Memorial Hermann Hospital; Hazim J. Safi, MD, McGovern Medical School at UTHealth, Houston, TX.)

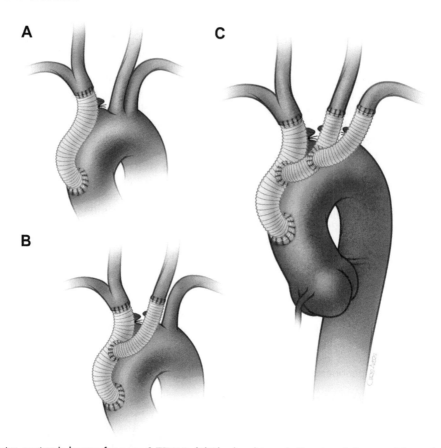

Fig. 3. Extra-anatomic bypass for zone 0 TEVAR. (*A*) The brachiocephalic artery is bypassed from the ascending aorta. (*B*) A bypass to the left common carotid artery is performed using the ascending aorta to brachiocephalic artery bypass as an inflow. (*C*) A bypass to the subclavian artery is added. (*Courtesy of* Chris Akers, MA, Memorial Hermann Hospital; Hazim J. Safi, MD, McGovern Medical School at UTHealth, Houston, TX.)

replaced with a graft because the ascending aorta greater than 4.0 cm is at risk for type A dissection.[26,27] Postoperative mortality is reported as 0% to 8%, and stroke is observed in 0% to 17%.[23,24,26,28] These numbers are comparable to the outcomes of isolated transsternal supra-aortic vessel bypasses reported by previous studies over the past 20 years.[29–31]

Zone 1 hybrid debranching arch repair is indicated for patients with distal arch abnormality whose proximal landing zone distal to the innominate artery is greater than 2 cm. Before TEVAR, revascularization of the left carotid (and left subclavian bypass) is performed. The bypass is usually performed by an extrathoracic approach using an 8-mm polytetrafluoroethylene or Dacron graft via anterior subplatysmal plane[20] or the retroesophageal route following planes between the buccopharyngeal fascia and the prevertebral fascia.[1,32] The retroesophageal path provides the shortest route and is well protected from injury because of the position of the graft deep in the neck. There are surgeons who prefer the transposition technique to avoid the use of prosthetic

material, in which the bypass is performed with sternotomy or hemisternotomy.[33] At the time of bypass, the proximal left carotid artery is ligated to prevent type II endoleak. The proximal left subclavian artery is similarly closed or plugged as needed. The endograft is then deployed via retrograde femoral access (**Fig. 5**). Postoperative mortality following zone 1 debranching TEVAR is 0% to 11% and stroke is 5% to 11%.[23,26,28]

The zone 2 deployment, covering the left subclavian artery, is often used in treating type B dissection or proximal descending aortic aneurysm. Indication for left subclavian artery revascularization in TEVAR remains controversial. A report from European Collaborators on Stent/Graft Techniques for Aortic Aneurysm Repair database[34] demonstrated that coverage of the left subclavian artery without revascularization increased the risk of postoperative paraplegia by nearly 4-fold. Stroke was also reported to be higher when the left subclavian artery was not revascularized, and other studies support these results.[34,35] To date, the Society of Vascular Surgery recommends routine preoperative revascularization of the left subclavian artery for elective

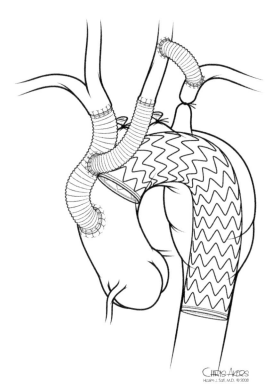

Fig. 4. Zone 0 hybrid TEVAR. The aortic arch aneurysm involving the transverse arch and the proximal descending aorta is repaired with extra-anatomic bypass and endografting. (*Courtesy of* Chris Akers, MA, Memorial Hermann Hospital; Hazim J. Safi, MD, McGovern Medical School at UTHealth, Houston, TX.)

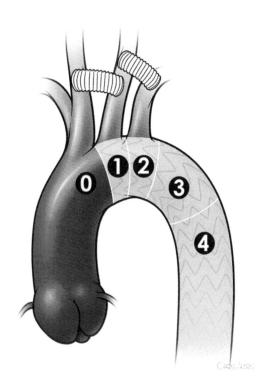

Fig. 5. Zone 1 hybrid TEVAR. (*Courtesy of* Chris Akers, MA, Memorial Hermann Hospital; Hazim J. Safi, MD, McGovern Medical School at UTHealth, Houston, TX.)

TEVAR with the left subclavian coverage,[36] especially in patients with the following circumstances: presence of patent left mammary to coronary artery bypass graft; functional left upper extremity arteriovenous fistula and planned long segmental coverage (>20 cm) of the descending aorta; absent right vertebral artery; infrarenal aortic operation; hypogastric artery occlusion; and presence of early aneurysmal disease where future therapy involving the distal thoracic aorta may be necessary (**Fig. 6**). Postoperative mortality and stroke following zone 2 TEVAR is reported as 0% to 3.4% and 3% to 8.7%, respectively.[28,37] Of note, these adverse events may be higher in the patients who underwent TEVAR on the same day of subclavian artery compared with those who received bypass procedures 30-day before TEVAR.[38]

TOTAL ENDOVASCULAR APPROACH
Parallel Stent Graft Technique

The parallel endograft technique (also known as snorkel or chimney technique), which was first used as a bailout procedure, has become an option to maintain blood flow to the vital branches within the sealing zone of the aortic stent graft

without the use of fenestrated or branched graft.[39] Briefly, a bare or covered stent is deployed into vital aortic branches parallel to the main aortic stent graft, between the aortic wall and the graft main body, so that the aortic stent is extended beyond the origin of the aortic branches. The parallel graft works as a functional branch of the stent graft. A recent review by Moulakakis and colleagues[40] (N = 124) demonstrated that primary delivery success was 99% (123 or 124) and perioperative mortality was 4.8% (6 of 124). However, the problem with parallel endograft techniques is type Ia endoleak, because the parallel stent graft may cause insufficient attachment of the graft body to the aortic wall.

Kanaoka and colleagues[1] recently reported high type Ia endoleak rate (26.9%, 14 of 38) after TEVAR and was a significant predictor for type Ia endoleak (OR: 5.3, 95% CI: 2.48–11.24, $P<.001$). Meanwhile, a European multicenter registry reported that type I endoleak was observed in 10.5% (10 of 95), and only half of the patients required reintervention (5.2%, 5 of 95).[41] A review of parallel endograft techniques used to treat juxtarenal or complex abdominal aortic aneurysm demonstrated that the type I endoleak rate increases with the number of the parallel devices used (1 parallel graft, 7%; 2 parallel grafts, 16%).[42] Thus, the endoleak rate

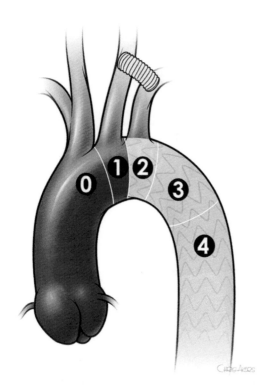

Fig. 6. Zone 2 hybrid repair. A bypass from the left common carotid to the left subclavian artery is performed. (*Courtesy of* Chris Akers, MA, Memorial Hermann Hospital; Hazim J. Safi, MD, McGovern Medical School at UTHealth, Houston, TX.)

may be improved by limiting the number of parallel endografts. It is also recommended to have the overlapping of the parallel endograft and the main graft by at least 2 to 3 cm to facilitate enough accommodation of the parallel graft and the main graft.[43] In addition, the stroke rate is often reported around 4% with the parallel endograft technique. This relatively high incidence is thought to be due to embolic stroke caused by the manipulation of the arch vessels. Nonetheless, the parallel endograft technique is a viable option for emergent or urgent cases in patients who are unfit for open surgical repair and as a bailout procedure in case of unplanned coverage.

Branched Endografts

There is no commercially available device available on the market yet in the United States. Two device systems with one branch are now being investigated in the United States. The Valiant Mona LSA stent graft system (Medtronic Inc, Santa Rosa, CA, USA) feasibility study showed promising results without mortality, major stroke, and endoleak requiring secondary interventions among all the 9 zone 2 deployments.[44] The GORE TAG Thoracic

Branch Endoprosthesis (W.L. Gore & Associates Inc, Newark, DE, USA) (**Fig. 7**) for zone 0 to 2 deployments is also undergoing an early feasibility study (**Fig. 8**). However, to date, no data are available. In addition, there are stent graft devices with 1 to 2 branches designed for zone 0 deployments being investigated outside the United States. Recently, a group from Europe and Japan reported outcomes of 55 patients using Cook Medical (Bloomington, IN, USA) inner branched arch endograft (2 inner branch gates) to treat aortic arch aneurysms in patients unfit for surgery.[45] Postoperative stroke was 16% and morality was 9% in this series. The mortality is satisfactory. However, the stroke rate remains relatively high. Also, both the early and the follow-up secondary procedure rates were nearly 10%. The other device based on the Bolton Relay NBS Plus (Bolton Medical, Sunrise, FL, USA) with 1/2 branches is being developed and has been used to treat patients in Europe (no data available). Mid-term and long-term outcomes are awaited to prove the safety and durability of these new devices.

In Situ Fenestration

In situ stent graft fenestration was first described by McWilliams and colleagues in 2004.[46] They used a stiff end of a guidewire followed by a needle and cutting balloon angioplasty. This technique seemed relatively simple, but it was later found that needle puncture caused tears in the expanded polytetrafluoroethylene (ePTFE)-based stent graft, and cutting the balloon resulted in significant fabric tears in both the ePTFE and the Dacron endografts.[47] Thus, in recent studies, laser or radiofrequency puncture has been used to create retrograde in situ fenestration during TEVAR.[48–50] These techniques are limited to zone 1 and 2 without the use of extracorporeal perfusion to maintain cerebral circulation[51] because they result in temporary occlusion of the covered supra-aortic branches. Briefly, for zone

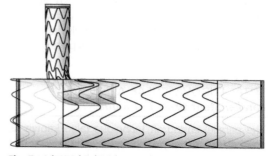

Fig. 7. A branched endovascular prosthesis (GORE TAG Thoracic Branch Endoprosthesis). (*Courtesy of* W. L. Gore & Associates, Inc, Newark, DE; with permission.)

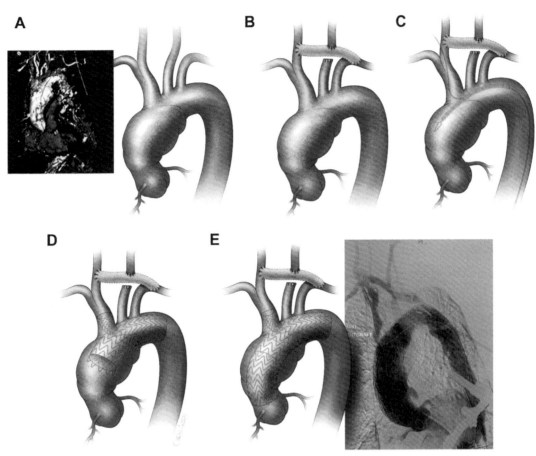

Fig. 8. Zone 0 hybrid TEVAR using a branched stent graft. (*A*) The transverse aortic arch aneurysm extends proximal to the ascending aorta. (*B*) A bypass from the right common carotid artery to the left common carotid and left subclavian artery is performed before the stent grafting. (*C*) A branched device is advanced from a femoral access. (*D*) The device is deployed to zone 0 with the branch in the brachiocephalic artery. (*E*) An additional stent graft is added proximally. The angiogram at the completion demonstrates the exclusion of the aneurysm with preserved flow to the supra-aortic vessels. (*Courtesy of* Chris Akers, MA, Memorial Hermann Hospital; Hazim J. Safi, MD, McGovern Medical School at UTHealth, Houston, TX.)

2, a guidewire is advanced to the origin of the left subclavian artery from the left brachial access, and the thoracic endograft is deployed across the left subclavian artery orifice. The guidewire is exchanged to the radiofrequency guidewire, and the graft is punctured using the "high" setting of the radiofrequency generator. The hole generated is dilated with an angioplasty balloon, and a covered stent is placed within the orifice. Both laser and radiofrequency fenestrations create relatively clear holes. The success of both of these techniques is highly dependent on the take-off angle of the left subclavian artery. An angle of 90° to the graft is ideal to create a clean, circular fenestration, whereas angles less than 30° will not allow the fenestration to be created.[52] The advantage of the radiofrequency device over the laser catheter is their availability. Radiofrequency wires are widely used for electrophysiologists and interventional radiologists. Thus, the device is available in most of the facilities without additional cost. However, the technical success was lower in the radiofrequency technique (60% vs 83%).[51,52] Further accumulation of data is required to evaluate the true value of both radiofrequency and laser fenestration techniques.

SUMMARY

Endovascular aortic repair to treat aortic arch abnormality has rapidly expanded in the last 2 decades. Surgeons now have options to treat patients who are poor candidates for open surgery. The devices and techniques should be tailored to the extension of the aortic abnormality and anatomy of the individuals. Recent studies demonstrate promising results with branched endografts, but one of the major drawbacks of the devices is that considerable time is required to prepare the custom-made graft, which may not be available for emergent or urgent cases. Introduction of commercially available devices is forthcoming. In addition, the risk of stroke following endovascular repair of the aortic arch remains as high as for conventional open surgery. Nonetheless, until the long-term outcomes become available, the indications of endovascular treatment should be carefully considered in patients with low risk for open surgical repair, especially in young patients with connective tissue disorders.

REFERENCES

1. Kanaoka Y, Ohki T, Maeda K, et al. Analysis of risk factors for early type I endoleaks after thoracic endovascular aneurysm repair. J Endovasc Ther 2017;24(1):89–96.
2. Criado FJ, McKendrick C, Criado FR. Technical solutions for common problems in TEVAR: managing access and aortic branches. J Endovasc Ther 2009; 16(Suppl 1):63–79.
3. Saleh HM, Inglese L. Combined surgical and endovascular treatment of aortic arch aneurysms. J Vasc Surg 2006;44(3):460–6.
4. Okita Y, Okada K, Omura A, et al. Total arch replacement using antegrade cerebral perfusion. J Thorac Cardiovasc Surg 2013;31(145):S63–71.
5. Nota H, Asai T, Suzuki T, et al. Risk factors for acute kidney injury in aortic arch surgery with selective cerebral perfusion and mild hypothermic lower body circulatory arrest. Interact Cardiovasc Thorac Surg 2014;19:955–61.
6. Leshnower BG, Kilgo PD, Chen EP. Total arch replacement using moderate hypothermic circulatory arrest and unilateral selective antegrade cerebral perfusion. J Thorac Cardiovasc Surg 2014;147:1488–92.
7. Estrera AL, Sandhu HK, Miller CC, et al. Repair of extensive aortic aneurysms: a single-center experience using the elephant trunk technique over 20 years. Ann Surg 2014;260:510–8.
8. Karck M, Chavan A, Hagl C, et al. The frozen elephant trunk technique: a new treatment for thoracic aortic aneurysms. J Thorac Cardiovasc Surg 2003;125(6):1550–3.
9. Liu ZG, Sun LZ, Chang Q, et al. Should the "elephant trunk" be skeletonized? Total arch replacement combined with stented elephant trunk implantation for Stanford type A aortic dissection. J Thorac Cardiovasc Surg 2006;131(1):107–13.
10. Pochettino A, Brinkman WT, Moeller P, et al. Antegrade thoracic stent grafting during repair of acute DeBakey I dissection prevents development of thoracoabdominal aortic aneurysms. Ann Thorac Surg 2009;88:482–90.
11. Borst HG, Walterbusch G, Schaps D. Extensive aortic replacement using "elephant trunk" prosthesis. Thorac Cardiovasc Surg 1983;31:37–40.
12. Kato M, Ohnishi K, Kaneko M, et al. New graft-implanting method for thoracic aortic aneurysm or dissection with a stented graft. Circulation 1996; 94(9 Suppl):II188–93.
13. Kato M, Kuratani T, Kaneko M, et al. The results of total arch graft implantation with open stent-graft placement for type A aortic dissection. J Thorac Cardiovasc Surg 2002;124:531–40.
14. Tsagakis K, Pacini D, Di Bartolomeo R, et al. Multicenter early experience with extended aortic repair in acute aortic dissection: is simultaneous descending stent grafting justified? J Thorac Cardiovasc Surg 2010;140(6 Suppl):S116–20.
15. Katayama A, Uchida N, Katayama K, et al. The frozen elephant trunk technique for acute type A aortic dissection: results from 15 years of experience. Eur J Cardiothorac Surg 2015;47:355–60.
16. Leontyev S, Tsagakis K, Pacini D, et al. Impact of clinical factors and surgical techniques on early outcome of patients treated with frozen elephant trunk technique by using EVITA open stent-graft: results of a multicentre study. Eur J Cardiothorac Surg 2016;49:660–6.
17. Shrestha M, Kaufeld T, Beckmann E, et al. Total aortic arch replacement with a novel 4-branched frozen elephant trunk prosthesis: single-center results of the first 100 patients. J Thorac Cardiovasc Surg 2016;152:148–59.
18. Buth J, Penn O, Tielbeek A, et al. Combined approach to stent-graft treatment of an aortic arch aneurysm. J Endovasc Ther 1998;5:329–32.
19. Kato M, Kaneko M, Kuratani T, et al. New operative method for distal aortic arch aneurysm: combined cervical branch bypass and endovascular stent-graft implantation. J Thorac Cardiovasc Surg 1999;117:832–4.
20. Shigemura N, Kato M, Kuratani T, et al. New operative method for acute type B dissection: left carotid artery–left subclavian artery bypass combined with endovascular stent-graft implantation. J Thorac Cardiovasc Surg 2000;120:406–8.
21. Mitchell RS, Ishimaru S, Ehrlich MP, et al. First international summit on thoracic aortic endografting: roundtable on thoracic aortic dissection as an indication for endografting. J Endovasc Ther 2002; 9(Suppl 2):II-98.
22. Fillinger MF, Greenberg RK, McKinsey JF, et al, Society for Vascular Surgery Ad Hoc Committee on TEVAR Reporting Standards. Reporting standards for thoracic endovascular aortic repair (TEVAR). J Vasc Surg 2010;52:1022–33.
23. Andersen ND, Williams JB, Hanna JM, et al. Results with an algorithmic approach to hybrid repair of the aortic arch. J Vasc Surg 2013;57:655–67.

24. Narita H, Komori K, Usui A, et al. Postoperative outcomes of hybrid repair in the treatment of aortic arch aneurysms. Ann Vasc Surg 2016;34:55–61.

25. Kuratani T, Sawa Y. Current strategy of endovascular aortic repair for thoracic aortic aneurysms. Gen Thorac Cardiovasc Surg 2010;58:393–8.

26. Bavaria J, Vallabhajosyula P, Moeller P, et al. Hybrid approaches in the treatment of aortic arch aneurysms: postoperative and midterm outcomes. J Thorac Cardiovasc Surg 2013;145:S85–90.

27. Williams JB, Andersen ND, Bhattacharya SD, et al. Retrograde ascending aortic dissection as an early complication of thoracic endovascular aortic repair. J Vasc Surg 2012;55:1255–62.

28. Yoshitake A, Hachiya T, Okamoto K, et al. Postoperative stroke after debranching with thoracic endovascular aortic repair. Ann Vasc Surg 2016;36:132–8.

29. Kieffer E, Sabatier J, Koskas F, et al. Atherosclerotic innominate artery occlusive disease: early and long-term results of surgical reconstruction. J Vasc Surg 1995;21:326–36.

30. Berguer R, Morasch MD, Kline RA. Transthoracic repair of innominate and common carotid artery disease: immediate and long-term outcome for 100 consecutive surgical reconstructions. J Vasc Surg 1998;27:34–41.

31. Rhodes JM, Cherry KJ Jr, Clark RC, et al. Aortic-origin reconstruction of the great vessels: risk factors of early and late complications. J Vasc Surg 2000;31:260–9.

32. Ozsvath KJ, Roddy SP, Darling RC, et al. Carotid-carotid crossover bypass: is it a durable procedure? J Vasc Surg 2003;37:582–5.

33. Czerny M, Weigang E, Sodeck G, et al. Targeting landing zone 0 by total arch rerouting and TEVAR: midterm results of a transcontinental registry. Ann Thorac Surg 2012;94:84–9.

34. Buth J, Harris PL, Hobo R, et al. Neurologic complications associated with endovascular repair of thoracic aortic pathology: incidence and risk factors. A study from the European Collaborators on Stent/Graft Techniques for Aortic Aneurysm Repair (EUROSTAR) registry. J Vasc Surg 2007;46:1103–11.

35. Patterson BO, Holt PJ, Nienaber C, et al. Management of the left subclavian artery and neurologic complications after thoracic endovascular aortic repair. J Vasc Surg 2014;60:1491–8.

36. Matsumura JS, Rizvi AZ. Left subclavian artery revascularization: Society for Vascular Surgery practice guidelines. J Vasc Surg 2010;52:65S–70S.

37. Kanaoka Y, Ohki T, Maeda K, et al. Multivariate analysis of risk factors of cerebral infarction in 439 patients undergoing thoracic endovascular aneurysm repair. Medicine (Baltimore) 2016;95:e3335.

38. Wilson JE, Galiñanes EL, Hu P, et al. Routine revascularization is unnecessary in the majority of patients requiring zone II coverage during thoracic endovascular aortic repair: a longitudinal outcomes study using United States Medicare population data. Vascular 2014;22:239–45.

39. Greenberg RK, Clair D, Srivastava S, et al. Should patients with challenging anatomy be offered endovascular aneurysm repair? J Vasc Surg 2003;38:990–6.

40. Moulakakis KG, Mylonas SN, Dalainas I, et al. The chimney-graft technique for preserving supra-aortic branches: a review. Ann Cardiothorac Surg 2013;2:339–46.

41. Bosiers MJ, Donas KP, Mangialardi N, et al. European Multicenter Registry for the Performance of the Chimney/Snorkel technique in the treatment of aortic arch pathologic conditions. Ann Thorac Surg 2016;101:2224–30.

42. Moulakakis KG, Mylonas SN, Avgerinos E, et al. The chimney graft technique for preserving visceral vessels during endovascular treatment of aortic pathologies. J Vasc Surg 2012;55:1497–503.

43. Lachat M, Frauenfelder T, Mayer D, et al. Complete endovascular renal and visceral artery revascularization and exclusion of a ruptured type IV thoracoabdominal aortic aneurysm. J Endovasc Ther 2010;17:216–20.

44. Roselli EE, Arko FR, Thompson MM, Valiant Mona LSA Trial Investigators. Results of the Valiant Mona LSA early feasibility study for descending thoracic aneurysms. J Vasc Surg 2015;62:1465–71.

45. Spear R, Haulon S, Ohki T, et al. Editor's choice–subsequent results for arch aneurysm repair with inner branched endografts. Eur J Vasc Endovasc Surg 2016;51:380–5.

46. McWilliams RG, Murphy M, Hartley D, et al. In situ stent-graft fenestration to preserve the left subclavian artery. J Endovasc Ther 2004;11:170–4.

47. Riga CV, Bicknell CD, Basra M, et al. In vitro fenestration of aortic stent-grafts: implications of puncture methods for in situ fenestration durability. J Endovasc Ther 2013;20:536–43.

48. Murphy EH, Dimaio JM, Dean W, et al. Endovascular repair of acute traumatic thoracic aortic transection with laser-assisted in-situ fenestration of a stent-graft covering the left subclavian artery. J Endovasc Ther 2009;16:457–63.

49. Ahanchi SS, Almaroof B, Stout CL, et al. In situ laser fenestration for revascularization of the left subclavian artery during emergent thoracic endovascular aortic repair. J Endovasc Ther 2012;19:226–30.

50. Leonard WT, Lindsay TF, Roche-Nagle G, et al. Radiofrequency in situ fenestration for aortic arch vessels during thoracic endovascular repair. J Endovasc Ther 2015;22:116–21.

Aortic Arch Pathology
Surgical Options for the Aortic Arch Replacement

Giorgio Zanotti, MD, Thomas Brett Reece, MD,
Muhammad Aftab, MD*

KEYWORDS

• Aortic arch • Aortic arch pathology • Ischemia • Aortic arch repair • Graft • Aortic arch surgery

KEY POINTS

• Aortic arch surgery remains one of the most technically challenging procedures in cardiac surgery.
• Arch surgery demands consideration of myocardial, brain, spinal cord, visceral organs and lower body protection.
• A better understanding of the effects of brain and systemic ischemia during circulatory arrest, refinements in brain and end-organ protection, use of antegrade cerebral perfusion and moderate hypothermia have made arch repair safer.
• Novel surgical approaches have revolutionized arch surgery.
• As endovascular technology and open surgical techniques evolve, aortic surgeons learn and incorporate these methods into routine practice.

INTRODUCTION

Intervention of the aortic arch remains one of the more technically challenging procedures in cardiac surgery. These procedures demand consideration of not only myocardial protection, but also brain protection, spinal cord, and the lower body. This article discusses the anatomic, pathologic, diagnostic, and procedural considerations applicable to optimal care for aortic arch patients.

ANATOMIC CONSIDERATIONS

The aortic arch, also called the transverse aortic arch, is the segment of the aorta providing the origins of the brachiocephalic vessels. The usual anatomy of the left-sided arch includes, from proximal to distal, the origin of the innominate or the brachiocephalic artery, which splits into the right subclavian and common carotid arteries,

followed by the left common carotid and finally the left subclavian artery. Important anomalies can affect the operative approach and must be recognized. The bovine arch is defined by the left common carotid arising from the innominate artery, and the vertebral artery can arise from the greater curve of the arch between the left common carotid and left subclavian arteries. Another common variation is called the anomalous right subclavian artery, commonly referred to as a Kommerrell's diverticulum. Careful review and understanding of the patient's anatomy and anomalies have to be taken into account for operative planning execution.

CLASSIFICATION OF AORTIC ARCH PATHOLOGY

For the consideration of surgical repair, aortic arch pathology can be broadly categorized into

Division of Cardiothoracic Surgery, Department of Surgery, Anschutz Medical Campus, University of Colorado, 12631 East 17th Avenue, Room 6602, Mail Stop C310, Aurora, CO 80045, USA
* Corresponding author. Division of Cardiothoracic Surgery, Department of Surgery, Anschutz Medical Campus, University of Colorado, 12631 East 17th Avenue, Room 6602, Mail Stop C310, Aurora, CO 80045.
E-mail address: muhammad.aftab@ucdenver.edu

Cardiol Clin 35 (2017) 367–385
http://dx.doi.org/10.1016/j.ccl.2017.03.006
0733-8651/17/© 2017 Elsevier Inc. All rights reserved.

arch aneurysm, acute or chronic dissection, penetrating ulcer, and intramural hematoma.

Aortic arch aneurysms are the most common arch pathology encountered by surgeons, which can be caused by a variety of conditions (**Table 1**). Arch aneurysms overall represent about 10% of the aneurysms involving the thoracic aorta. These are most commonly caused by chronic aortic dissection (53%), followed by atherosclerosis (29%), and all other etiologies (19%).[1] As such, most of the data available regarding treatment indications and outcomes are drawn from patients affected by chronic dissection with aneurysmal degeneration of the arch. Other causative factors include genetically triggered connective tissue diseases, infection, and trauma (see **Table 1**). Isolated aortic arch aneurysms, presenting as localized saccular outpouchings of the arch are quite uncommon. Most of the arch aneurysms involve the contiguous segments of the aorta including ascending and or descending thoracic aorta.

Intramural hematoma, penetrating ulcer, and aortic dissection are a heterogeneous subset with the potential for evolution from one into another and represent the minority of arch disease.

DIAGNOSIS AND ASSESSMENT OF THE AORTIC ARCH PATHOLOGY

Aortic aneurysm is generally defined as permanent dilation of a segment of aorta that is at least 50% greater than its normal diameter. In healthy adults, aortic diameters usually do not exceed 40 mm at the root, which is the largest segment of the vessel. The aorta then gradually tapers distally and its size is influenced by a variety of factors including age, sex, height, weight, and blood pressure.[2–5] Aging is associated with a physiologic rate of enlargement of 0.9 mm in men and 0.7 mm in women, every decade.[4]

Most arch aneurysms are asymptomatic and, as such, are usually discovered incidentally. However, patients with arch aneurysm can present with compressive symptoms to adjacent organs such as hoarseness, dysphagia, lower respiratory tract infections, chest pain, and upper body edema (superior vena cava syndrome). Dissections involving the aortic arch can present with symptoms of brain malperfusion such as syncope, transient ischemic attack, or stroke.

When suspecting aortic arch pathology, the assessment of each patient should be aimed at understanding the lamented complaints, interpreting physical findings that may suggest impaired perfusion such as asymmetric brachiocephalic and distal pulses, and an abnormal neurologic examination. Ascertaining an individual cardiovascular risk profile and gathering a family history of aneurysms or dissections and sudden death are tantamount for assessing need for aggressiveness of intervention. From this global evaluation, the physician will determine the pretest probability for the presence of arch pathology and, therefore, will select the most appropriate test to probe the initial working diagnosis.

Imaging remains the primary diagnostic tool for arch pathology. In particular, the preferred modality allows the visualization of the entire aorta in a comprehensive manner. Precise measurement of aortic arch aneurysm diameter can be challenging because the axial images through the aortic arch produce an oblong rather than a circular contour (**Fig. 1**). Furthermore, measuring the long axis contour is misleading because this does not truly represent the aortic arch aortic diameter.

From the imaging standpoint, a few key points need to be emphasized (see **Fig. 1**; **Fig. 2**):

1. The aortic arch is a complex, 3-dimensional structure; therefore, a standardized measurement technique is critical to detect true

---

Table 1
Etiology of aortic arch aneurysm

Etiology	Defect	Disease
Degenerative	Cystic medial degeneration	Atherosclerosis
	Spontaneous rupture of vasa vasora or atherosclerotic plaque	Intramural hematoma
	Ulceration of arteriosclerotic plaque	Penetrating arteriosclerotic ulcer
Connective tissue disorder	FNB1 gene mutation	Marfan syndrome
	TGFβ receptor 1 and 2, TGFβ, and SMAD gene mutations	Loeys-Dietz syndrome (type 1–4)
	Type III collagen synthesis	Ehlers-Danlos type IV
Infected	*Staphylococcus aureus, S epidermidis, Salmonella, Treponemapallidum*	Mycotic aneurysm

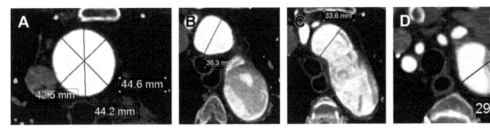

Fig. 1. Aortic arch diameter assessment based on axial images (*A–D*). The aortic arch diameter is measured just proximal to the take off of the innominate artery (*A*), between innominate and left common carotid artery (*B*), between the left common carotid and the left subclavian (*C*) and at the isthmus (*D*).

changes in size and shape. The aortic arch diameter should be measured at the take off of the innominate artery, between the innominate and left common carotid artery, between left common carotid and the left subclavian and at the isthmus.

2. Measurements must be taken perpendicular to the axis of centerline of flow. When this is not possible, the smallest diameter more reliably represents the true size of the vessel.

3. Serial examinations using the same imaging technique with side-by-side comparisons are the most reliable way to detect interval changes in the aortic diameter. Because the interobserver variability of computed tomography (CT) scan measurements is 5 mm, changes in diameter of less than 5 mm may not be clinically relevant and, therefore, serial evaluation is crucial.[6,7]

4. Finally, although there is no consensus as to whether measurements should include the

aortic wall or not, the current prognostic data are inclusive of the aortic wall.[8] Therefore, CT scan measurements typically are obtained from outer wall to outer wall, even if the presence of thrombus may significantly affect sizing.[9]

CT angiogram plays a pivotal role in the diagnosis and management planning of arch pathology and it is the most widely used diagnostic study for aortic arch pathology. For best image acquisition, electrocardiogram gating is crucial. Also, contrast-enhanced images are recommended for a complete assessment of the aortic wall pathology (specifically for dissection, intramural hematoma, and penetrating ulcer). Advantages of CT angiogram include its widespread use, the possibility to obtain 3-dimensional reconstruction and perform image manipulation with advanced software to minimize the effects of "off-axis" measurements and short time required for image acquisition. Some of its disadvantages include administration

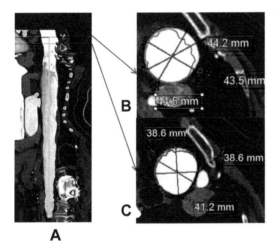

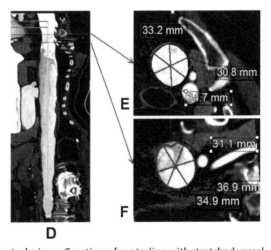

Fig. 2. Aortic arch diameter assessment using the centerline technique. Creation of centerline with stretched vessel view (*A, D*) allows viewing of aortic arch in cross-sectional planes perpendicular to the aorta. The aortic diameter can be either automatically calculated by the software or manual measurements could be performed in case of any interference by calcium or thrombus. The diameters of selected segments of aortic arch orthogonal to the centerline of flow (*A, D*) are shown, just proximal to the take off of the innominate artery (*B*), between innominate and left common carotid artery (*C*), between the left common carotid and the left subclavian (*E*) and at the isthmus (*F*).

of iodinated intravenous contrast and exposure to radiations.

MRI and magnetic resonance angiography have the ability to provide precise details on the aortic wall and lumen and the relationship of the aneurysm to the arch branch vessels, as well as flow through the true and false lumens in arch dissections. Also, freedom from iodinated intravenous contrast administration and lack of radiations make it a particularly attractive modality for serial follow-up imaging. However, the long time required for data acquisition and the nonimmediate availability render the MRI not as widespread.

Aortography use in arch pathology imaging is almost always limited to intraoperative imaging during stenting procedures. Inability to assess the aortic wall, invasiveness, and not immediate availability made contrast-enhanced gated CT angiogram the gold standard in aortic arch imaging.

In our practice, we use 3-dimensional imaging software (Aquarius iNtuition version 4.4; TeraRecon Inc., San Mateo, CA) to analyze the aorta from the raw data provided by contrast enhanced CT imaging. All the CT imaging studies are performed with 1-mm thick slices allowing a consistent and reproducible 3-dimensional analysis by the TeraRecon software. A centerline is constructed from the aortic root to the bifurcation of aorta or even distally, as needed. The diameters of all of the aortic segments are measured perpendicular to the centerline and all the lengths are measured along the same centerline.

SURGICAL INDICATIONS: AMERICAN HEART ASSOCIATION AND EUROPEAN SOCIETY OF CARDIOLOGY GUIDELINES

Arch aneurysms are repaired in a preventative manner to avoid complications such as dissection, aneurysm rupture, and death. Recommendations for surgical intervention in arch pathology are looser than other aortic segments. The lack of stringent criteria for intervention stems from the paucity of data on arch disease. Furthermore, the majority of the arch aneurysms are contiguous with aneurysmal degeneration of the ascending and descending thoracic aorta. Hence, the natural history of arch aneurysms is not well-understood because they tend to be intervened on based on disparate, but adjacent, pathology.

The risks of aorta-related complications are also mitigated by a higher risk of neurologic complications intrinsic to the manipulation of the brachiocephalic vessels for the aortic arch repair. Based on the current literature, the risk of stroke is reportedly 5% to 10%.[10–13] For this reason, the decision to operate on the arch should be based on the preoperative risk profile for surgery, risk of aortic complications for any given individual, the need for adjunctive cardiac surgery procedures, the presence of symptoms, and the anatomy of the entire thoracic aorta, given that arch aneurysm is often associated to enlargement of the ascending and/or descending aorta.

Current North American treatment guidelines make several scenario-based recommendations (class IIa, level of evidence B) on arch interventions, which are summarized in **Table 2**.[14] The limitation to these guidelines is that the approach to repair the aortic arch is generally driven by the extent of disease of the adjacent ascending or descending aorta.

Table 2
Recommendations on the surgical intervention for the aortic arch aneurysm based on American College of Cardiology/American Heart Association practice guidelines (class IIa, level of evidence: B)

Type of Arch Replacement	Segment of Arch Enlarged	Recommendations
Partial	Proximal	When ascending aneurysm extending into proximal arch
Complete	Distal	As initial part (elephant trunk) of staged repair of descending aorta aneurysm extending into the distal arch
	Whole	1. Diameter ≥55 mm, in low-risk, asymptomatic patients 2. If acute dissection, when arch is dilated or major intimal destruction

Data from Hiratzka LF, Bakris GL, Beckman JA, et al. 2010 ACCF/AHA/AATS/ACR/ASA/SCA/SCAI/SIR/STS/SVM guidelines for the diagnosis and management of patients with Thoracic Aortic Disease: a report of the American College of Cardiology Foundation/American Heart Association Task Force on Practice Guidelines, American Association for Thoracic Surgery, American College of Radiology, American Stroke Association, Society of Cardiovascular Anesthesiologists, Society for Cardiovascular Angiography and Interventions, Society of Interventional Radiology, Society of Thoracic Surgeons, and Society for Vascular Medicine. Circulation 2010;121:e266–369.

The 2014 European Society of Cardiology guidelines[15] provide similar recommendations regarding surgical intervention (arch diameter ≥55 mm). In addition, there is an emphasis on the presence of symptoms—surgery should be considered in patients with symptoms or signs of compression (dysphagia, dyspnea, voice character changes)—or the need for concomitant cardiac surgical procedures. No clear guidelines exist regarding the surgical treatment of isolated, asymptomatic intramural hematoma, or penetrating ulcer of the arch.

Based on these guidelines, our practice is to perform total aortic arch replacement in low-risk, asymptomatic patients with isolated arch aneurysm, when either the aortic diameter exceeds 5.5 cm or the aneurysmal growth rate is greater than 0.5 cm per year. Patients with saccular aneurysms pose a particular threat of complications owing to rapid growth; hence, we tend to intervene earlier in these patients. For patients with ascending aortic aneurysm and limited proximal arch involvement, we perform extended hemiarch/partial arch replacement in addition to the ascending aortic repair. Total arch replacement is, however, preferred in patients with chronic dissection and aneurysms with involvement of the proximal descending thoracic aorta. In particular, these patients are candidates for classic or frozen elephant trunk repair to address distal thoracic aortic pathology. Moreover, total arch replacement is performed in patients with symptomatic arch aneurysms regardless of the diameter, provided that the patient has an acceptable life expectancy. Although the asymptomatic patient with connective tissue disorders were not discussed in the guidelines, we tend to perform elective repair in patients free from symptoms with ascending aortic aneurysm and arch involvement and an aortic diameter of 4.0 to 4.5 cm, depending on the particular connective tissue disorder.

SURGICAL TREATMENT

Surgical repair of aortic arch is one of the most challenging procedures in cardiothoracic surgery. This is mainly because, to accomplish a total arch repair, blood flow to both brain and downstream end organs is interrupted.

Historical Perspective

The inception of aortic arch repair surgery dates back to the early 1950s, shortly preceded by critical bench work on the effects of organ hypothermia[16] and aortic cross-clamping.[17] The pioneering clinical work on aneurysmorrhaphy and graft interposition on the descending aorta carried out by Gross laid the ground work for subsequent aortic arch repairs.[18]

In 1952, Cooley and DeBakey[19] reported their initial experience on resection of sacciform, syphilitic aneurysms of the arch by lateral resection and suturing on a beating heart. In 1954, the same authors reported the first resection and grafting of a segment of the arch after traumatic transaction of the isthmus,[20] representing the first clinical application of hypothermia and aortic cross-clamping in aortic arch surgery. DeBakey and Cooley reported the first successful repair of transverse aortic arch in 1957 using a homograft. They also used an early form of antegrade cerebral perfusion (ACP) to perform this procedure.[21] In 1964, Borst and associates[22] used deep hypothermia along with circulatory arrest to repair a fistula between the arch and the pulmonary artery secondary to a gunshot wound. In 1975, Griepp and coworkers[23] described their experience with the use of deep hypothermic circulatory arrest for total arch replacement with great reduction in mortality and neurologic morbidity. In 1986, Guilmet and associates[24] published their experience with selective, ACP. They found that cerebral perfusion via the carotid arteries at 12°C would allow longer periods of deep circulatory arrest times while avoiding profound hypothermia core body temperatures. Subsequent developments that paved the way to modern arch surgery led to improved neurologic protection and optimized management of the brachiocephalic vessels. This, in turn, allowed minimizing hemorrhage and circulatory arrest time. Currently, arch repair can be accomplished using a traditional open surgical technique, a combination of both open and endovascular procedures, also called hybrid arch repair and total endovascular arch repair techniques. The last 2 techniques are typically used in high-risk patients to further reduce the perioperative morbidity and mortality.

OPEN SURGICAL ARCH REPAIR: MANAGEMENT OF ARCH VESSELS

Reconstitution of blood flow into the brachiocephalic vessels is a critical step in aortic arch reconstruction. Several strategies are in the armamentarium of the aortic surgeon.

Partial Arch Repair

Aneurysm involving only the proximal portion of transverse arch are usually treated with a partial arch repair, also called an extended hemiarch. It is a less complex repair, because it does not require reattachment of arch vessels. This technique is used in patients with fusiform ascending aortic aneurysm extending into the proximal portion of the arch, whereas the distal arch is normal in size. In the hemiarch approach, the surgical graft is beveled to replace the proximal portion of the aortic arch along the lesser curvature.

Total Arch Replacement: "Island Patch Technique"

In patients with the extensive arch aneurysms requiring the total replacement of aortic arch, the 3 arch vessels can be harvested as part of a large, single patch of aortic wall and are reimplanted with a single anastomosis on the dome of the prosthetic arch graft, typically during a period of hypothermic circulatory arrest. This technique was originally introduced to minimize circulatory arrest time, and simplify reimplantation of and minimize manipulation of the brachiocephalic vessels. This technique does not, however, allow treatment of chronic dissection involving the residual "island" tissue and the arch branches. Also, it poses a risk of anastomotic pseudoaneurysms because the suture line involves diseased aorta. In fact, "island patch" aneurysm has been reported, particularly in patients with connective tissue disorders.

Because of these limitations, in the past decades, 2 newer techniques have essentially replaced the island patch technique. These include the trifurcated or Y-graft technique[25] and the integrated, 4-branched arch graft technique.[26] These techniques allow a shorter duration of deep hypothermic circulatory arrest and provide an opportunity for the bilateral ACP for cerebral protection.

Total Arch Replacement: Y-Graft Technique

Spielvogel and colleagues[25] initially proposed trifurcated Y-graft technique in 2002. This technique has been adopted widely with some modifications to the various patterns of Y grafts for the arch reconstruction based on the individual patients' pathology (**Figs. 3** and **4**). For this purpose, either a commercially available prefabricated Y-graft can be used or surgeons, on the back table, can construct a double Y-branched graft by suture anastomosing the 2 limbs of an 8-mm graft to a main trunk of a 12-mm graft, or 2 limbs of 10-mm grafts to 14-mm main body graft, at a 45° angle.

The implementation of this technique is made possible by the extensive network of collaterals connecting the 3 arch vessels and those with the upper and lower body. This allows for a brief period of occlusion of 1 or 2 brachiocephalic vessels while the others perfuse their territory. Briefly, cardiopulmonary bypass is established with either /innominate artery or femoral inflow, moderate hypothermia is induced and the arch vessels are

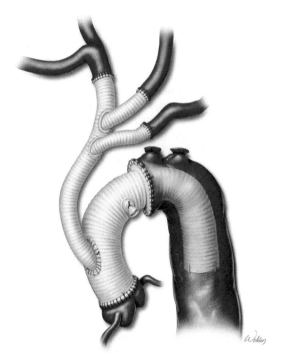

Fig. 3. The Y-graft technique of aortic arch replacement with an elephant trunk. (*Courtesy of* Baylor College of Medicine, Houston, TX; with permission.)

serially disconnected and reconstructed from the innominate to the subclavian using a trifurcated arch graft. The perfusion side arm of the trifurcated graft can be used to establish bilateral antegrade cerebral reperfusion after reconstruction of the arch vessels. This technique allows for complete arch replacement without the need for global circulatory arrest, thus avoiding potential ischemic injury to the spine and abdominal organs. Also, the open distal anastomosis can be carried out more proximally and unhurried and therefore considered to facilitate a more hemostatic suture line. The branch vessels are reanastomosed more distally, minimizing manipulation of diseased, proximal segments. The common stem of the trifurcated graft is then anastomosed to the proximal aspect of the ascending deployment in the arch in case a frozen elephant trunk is part of the plan.

Four-Branched or Branch-Last Arch Replacement

Kazui and colleagues[26] described this classical technique for total arch replacement. Using a commercially available 4-branched graft, an open distal aortic anastomosis is performed during deep, hypothermic circulatory arrest. The distal aortic anastomosis can be performed

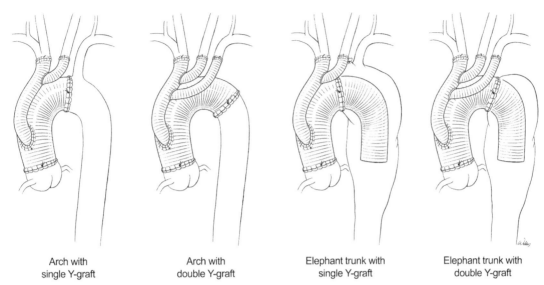

| Arch with | Arch with | Elephant trunk with | Elephant trunk with |
| single Y-graft | double Y-graft | single Y-graft | double Y-graft |

Fig. 4. Different configurations of the Y-graft technique for replacing the aortic arch. These include the arch with a single Y-graft, the arch with a double Y-graft, the elephant trunk with a single Y-graft, and the elephant trunk with a double Y-graft. (*Courtesy of* Baylor College of Medicine, Houston, TX; with permission.)

with or without cerebral perfusion. Antegrade systemic perfusion is resumed via a side branch of the arch graft, and systemic rewarming is initiated. Next the proximal aortic anastomosis is performed followed by myocardial reperfusion. Last, the brachiocephalic vessels are anastomosed to the graft beginning from the left subclavian artery moving proximal to the innominate artery. The advantage of using 4-branched grafts over the island technique is that it allows reimplantation of the brachiocephalic vessels last, therefore minimizing myocardial ischemia time. Also, no portion of the aneurysmal arch wall is part of the anastomoses. Hence, no residual diseased aortic tissue is left in place to cause formation of psudoaneurysms. This technique can be performed via both median sternotomy and left thoracotomy although the former reduces the risk of pulmonary complications from lung manipulation and the risk of recurrent laryngeal nerve injury. The neo-arch can be excised (exclusion technique) or wrapped by the native aortic wall left in situ (inclusion technique), although this is associated with increased risk of bleeding[27] and retained clot around the neo-arch. The interpretation of postoperative CT scan findings will need to take into consideration the surgical technique adopted.

MANAGEMENT OF DISTAL ARCH AND PROXIMAL DESCENDING AORTIC DISEASE
Elephant Trunk Technique

In patients with extensive aneurysms or dissections, where the distal arch pathology continues into the descending aorta, the surgical repair is performed in 2 stages. This is because the proximal aortic repair needs a different surgical exposure than the one for distal repair. In these patients, the decision to first repair the proximal or distal aortic segment is primarily based on symptoms, size of the aneurysm, and the need for additional cardiac procedures.

The classic elephant trunk procedure, first described by Borst and colleagues in 1983,[28] involves the repair of proximal aorta first with the extension of the arch repair beyond the aortic isthmus with an elephant trunk. The standard elephant trunk is a free-floating, 10-cm extension of the arch vascular graft past the distal arch anastomosis into the proximal descending aorta onto which either a stent graft or a conventional prosthetic conduit will be connected to at the time of the descending aorta repair via a left-sided thoracotomy or endovascular approach (**Fig. 5**). Essentially, the first stage of the elephant trunk procedure sets up the stage for a second stage, namely, completion replacement of the descending aorta. This technique simplifies the procedure by avoiding dissection of the distal arch in a reoperative field and therefore minimizes the chances of injury to the pulmonary artery, esophagus, and recurrent laryngeal nerve. It also facilitates the second stage procedure by decreasing the cross-clamp time and improving hemostasis owing to a graft-to-graft anastomosis, rather than a challenging distal arch to graft anastomosis. It also abrogates the need of circulatory arrest, which would be required in cases where the proximal aorta is large and

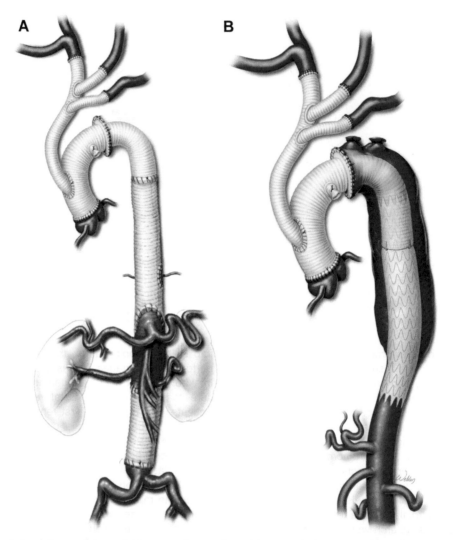

Fig. 5. Depiction of second-stage elephant trunk procedure: (*A*) Open elephant trunk completion and (*B*) Endovascular elephant trunk completion. (*Courtesy of* Baylor College of Medicine, Houston, TX; with permission.)

cannot be clamped to perform a safe anastomosis. Last, it provides a stable proximal landing zone in case a second stage, endovascular, elephant trunk completion repair is planned (in patients with the suitable anatomy).

A recent technical advancement to the elephant trunk procedure is the introduction of a "skirted" of "collared" arch graft. This is particularly helpful in patients where there is a substantial size discrepancy between the distal aortic arch and the arch graft. The skirt can be trimmed to match to the size of the aneurysm and a tension-free distal anastomosis can be performed. This simplifies the first stage procedure by minimizing the chances of distal anastomotic pseudoaneurysm and facilitates in optimal surgical hemostasis.

Reverse Elephant Trunk Technique

In extensive thoracic aortic aneurysms, where the descending thoracic or thoracoabdominal segment is symptomatic or disproportionately larger than the proximal ascending/arch aorta, the distal aortic repair is usually performed first. To facilitate the staged repair in such patients, an ingenious modification to the elephant trunk procedure is the "reversed elephant trunk technique," initially described by Carrel and Althaus and their colleagues.[29,30] They applied the elephant trunk principle, with a bidirectional approach, to distal thoracic aortic replacement. In reverse elephant trunk procedure, the aortic graft is invaginated within itself, like an intussusception in the proximal portion of the descending aorta distal to the left subclavian artery.[29,30] For the second staged proximal aortic operation, the invaginated elephant trunk segment is used to replace the aortic arch, thus eliminating the need for a distal anastomosis.

An inherent limitation to the open elephant trunk procedure is its staged nature. Usually, there is a 4- to 8-week interval between stages for the optimal postoperative recovery. These patients are at the risk of aneurysm rupture between the stages. The interval between the staged procedures can be shortened or second stage can be performed during the same hospitalization in symptomatic patients, patients with unreliable follow-up or the ones living in remote places where immediate medical care is not available in case of aneurysm rupture.

Frozen Elephant Trunk Procedure

The frozen elephant trunk technique was introduced in 1996 as a modification of standard elephant trunk procedure to treat the patients with extensive aortic aneurysms and chronic dissections involving the aortic arch and the distal aorta.[31] Using this technique, a median sternotomy is performed. After initiating the hypothermic circulatory arrest a stent graft is deployed into distal arch/proximal descending aorta. This is performed under direct vision through the transected aortic arch in an antegrade fashion. In the United States, the stent graft is suture secured into the arch proximally and affixed "frozen" into the descending thoracic aorta distally. Outside of the United States, various hybrid stent grafts are available, which further simplify the frozen elephant trunk procedure. The remaining surgical repair of ascending aorta and aortic arch is then performed in a standard fashion. The frozen elephant trunk technique simplifies the conventional elephant trunk operation, which is primarily a 2-stage procedure, into a 1-stage repair of extended aortic aneurysms in selected patients with similar operative mortality and greatly facilitates the subsequent distal aortic repair in others. In the frozen elephant trunk technique, the stent graft positioned into the distal aorta sufficiently promotes false lumen thrombosis to facilitate subsequent aortic remodeling in aortic dissections. Similarly, resolution of the nonperfused segment occurs after complete exclusion of the aneurysms. The surgical strategy is tailored specifically to address individual pathology based on each patient's aortic anatomy.

OUTCOMES OF TOTAL ARCH REPLACEMENT SURGERY

A precise representation of outcomes after total arch repair is virtually impossible given the heterogeneity of the aortic conditions (complicated, acute dissection vs chronic, atherosclerotic aneurysm vs reoperative surgery in the setting of chronic arch dissection) leading to surgery. Furthermore, the number of aortic segments involved by the disease that require treatment, concomitant procedures performed along with the relatively low number of cases performed annually even at specialized aortic centers makes the comparison of open arch repair outcomes even more challenging.

According to the most recent series of total arch replacement, in-hospital mortality ranges from 5% to 16%[10–13,32] and seems to be strongly correlated with cardiopulmonary bypass time, myocardial ischemia time, and circulatory arrest time.[13] The reported incidence of stroke is 5% to 10%,[10–13,32] but it becomes as high as 14% when there is dissection involving the arch vessels.[10] The occurrence of spinal cord injury rate is about 5% with a linear correlation with circulatory arrest time.[11–13] The overall 5-year survival is about 70%.[11,13,33] These results are representative of both conventional open arch replacement as well as hybrid arch techniques.

In short, total arch replacement surgery is a highly complex and technically challenging procedure. However, this can be accomplished with low mortality and good long-term outcomes in experienced hands and with a surgical plan individually tailored to each patient.

THE BUFFALO TRUNK TECHNIQUE OF TOTAL AORTIC ARCH REPLACEMENT

The basic tenets of our current approach to total aortic arch replacement include Innominate or axillary artery cannulation, use of moderate hypothermia with ACP, 4-branched graft technique with or without frozen elephant trunk, open distal anastomosis, and early body perfusion after distal anastomosis to minimize the systemic ischemia.

The innominate artery is our preferred cannulation site for the arterial inflow for cardiopulmonary bypass and selective ACP during circulatory arrest. A 10-mm Dacron side graft is anastomosed to the innominate artery in an end-to-side fashion after applying a side clamp (**Fig. 6**). The safety and effectiveness of innominate artery cannulation for proximal aortic surgery has been reported previously.[34] Some advantages include avoiding an additional surgical incision and local complications from surgical exposure of axillary artery, such as injury to the brachial plexus, dissection of the friable axillary artery, arm claudication, and ischemia. We tend to reserve right axillary cannulation for patients where the innominate artery

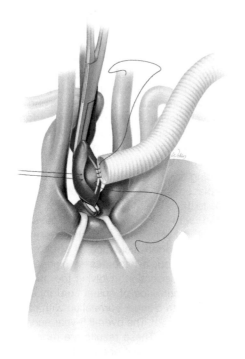

Fig. 6. Innominate artery annulation used for cardio-pulmonary bypass inflow and antegrade cerebral perfusion. After 1 to 1.5 mg/kg of heparin, a partial occluding clamp is applied on the innominate artery and a 10-mm graft is anastomosed to the artery in an end-to-side manner. (*Courtesy of* Baylor College of Medicine, Houston, TX; with permission.)

anatomy is not favorable, such as aortic dissection involving the innominate artery, significant atherosclerosis, or aneurysm of the vessel. Also, for high-risk reoperative sternotomies, where the vital mediastinal structures are densely plastered to the back of sternum, the axillary artery is our preferred access site. Femoral cannulation is usually reserved for the emergent situations. The arterial line of the bypass circuit is Y-ed in the beginning of the procedure, to establish systemic perfusion immediately after our open distal anastomosis using the side arm or the 4-branched graft.

After median sternotomy and opening the pericardium, the patient is fully heparinized. The right atrium is usually cannulated, and cardiopulmonary bypass is instituted.

We monitor brain perfusion by measuring cerebral oximetry using near-infrared spectroscopy and intraoperative electroencephalography. After establishing the cardiopulmonary pass, and while the patient is being actively cooled, we complete the remaining dissection of supraaortic arch

vessels, namely, the left common carotid and left subclavian arteries. At this point, the aorta can be clamped and the heart is arrested. The heart is usually protected using cold Del Nido cardioplegia. To optimize the myocardial protection, additional doses of cardioplegia are given after 60 to 90 minutes of initial induction dose (1000 mL) and then every 30 minutes (500 mL) thereafter in either retrograde or antegrade fashion directly through the coronary artery ostia. At this point, any of the proximal aortic or cardiac procedure including root replacement, valvular replacement/repair, or coronary revascularization can be performed.

After attaining the adequate cooling based on nasopharyngeal temperature of 24°C and or electroencephalography silence, bypass flows are reduced to 10 to 15 mL/kg/min and the innominate and left common carotid arteries are snared and modified circulatory arrest is initiated. At this point, the aortic clamp, if already applied, can be removed. The ascending aorta and arch are opened. The head is cooled into a cooling helmet. We usually deliver unilateral ACP through the innominate or axillary artery. Special attention is paid to maintaining an adequate bilateral hemispheric perfusion based on electroencephalographic monitoring and baseline near-infrared spectroscopy. ACP flows are adjusted to maintain the oximetry closer to baseline and pressure in the left arm is maintained at around 50 to 60 mm Hg. A balloon-tipped cannula can be used through the ostia of left common carotid artery to provide bilateral ACP, in the rare occasion of persistent left brain malperfusion despite the flows adjustments. The aortic aneurysm is resected and arch branches are mobilized and trimmed, leaving a button of aortic tissue for the individual bypasses. Next, the distal aorta for open distal anastomosis is prepared. Our preferred site for distal anastomosis is between the left subclavian and left carotid arteries. Four vessels branched graft with elephant trunk or a skirted elephant trunk graft can be used.

In case of extensive aneurysms, where the elephant trunk technique is required for subsequent distal aortic repair, we carefully insert the elephant trunk into the distal aorta. In patients with chronic dissections, it is carefully positioned into the true lumen. Occasionally, if the distal aortic dissection is complex, intravascular ultrasound imaging is used to ensure the access into the true aortic lumen.

We have developed a modified frozen elephant trunk technique where we deploy the endovascular stent graft, in an antegrade fashion, inside the classic elephant trunk graft already positioned into the aorta, thus combining both classic and frozen elephant trunk techniques, called the buffalo trunk technique. This method is essentially our modified version of the arch frozen elephant trunk grafts, which are currently not commercially available in the United States. Our distal anastomosis consists of a sandwich of (from inside of the aortic lumen outward) a frozen elephant trunk endograft, surgical elephant trunk graft, native distal aorta, and a strip of felt of bovine pericardium. This technique provides the benefits of frozen elephant trunk with distal aortic remodeling in patients with chronic dissection, avoiding occasional complications of the classic elephant trunk, such as graft kinking and malperfusion. This technique also ensures that the elephant trunk is positioned well in the true lumen, promotes true lumen expansion, false lumen thrombosis, and eventually provides a stable proximal landing zone for either distal endovascular or open aortic repair. Reconstruction of the left subclavian artery is performed next, because this anastomosis can be challenging. Sometimes a left carotid to subclavian bypass can be performed a few days before the total arch repair, which enables to move the distal aortic anastomosis more proximally. Some of the benefits of this approach include avoiding the left recurrent laryngeal nerve injury and ease of surgical hemostasis.

After the distal aortic and left subclavian anastomosis, the side branch of the graft is connected to an already Y-ed cardiopulmonary bypass circuit. The proximal graft is clamped and corporeal perfusion is reestablished. The remaining procedure is performed while both brain and systemic perfusion are maintained through separate systems. Systemic rewarming is initiated after 5 minutes of reestablishing systemic perfusion. Next, the side branches of 4-branched graft are trimmed and left common carotid and innominate arteries are anastomosed. Once arch reconstruction is completed, the grafts are carefully de-aired and clamps are removed. At this point, the remaining parts of any additional cardiovascular procedures can be completed. Next, the proximal aortic anastomosis is fashioned and coronary perfusion is restored (**Fig. 7**).

AORTIC ARCH ANOMALIES AND TECHNICAL CONSIDERATIONS

As mentioned, the arch anatomy requires careful consideration. The branch anatomy and sidedness of the arch should be evaluated carefully. In 5% of patients, both the innominate and left common carotid arteries share a common and slightly enlarged single ostium called the bovine aortic arch. The

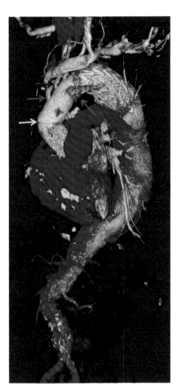

Fig. 7. The buffalo trunk technique of total aortic arch replacement. Volume-rendered 3-dimensional computed tomography reconstruction after total arch repair with frozen elephant trunk. The arrows depict proximal anastomosis (*yellow arrow*) and bypass grafts to innominate artery (*red arrow*), left common carotid artery (*blue arrow*), and left subclavian artery (*green arrow*). The distal anastomosis (*orange arrow*) incorporates the stent graft as frozen elephant trunk in the proximal descending aorta.

most important need for recognition with a bovine arch is that the single trunk cannot be occluded without understanding that the entire cerebral circulation arises from this take off. For the arch replacement, bovine trunk vessels can be either reimplanted as a single patch or 2 separate bypass grafts. Similarly, in rare occasions, a large left vertebral artery originates directly from the greater curvature of the aortic arch between the left common carotid and the left subclavian arteries. This can be implanted directly into the bypass graft of either left common carotid artery or left subclavian artery at the time of arch replacement.

Special attention should be paid to the presence of an aberrant right subclavian artery originating from the normal left-sided arch. This is the most common arch malformation with an incidence of 0.5% to 2.0%. In these cases, the right common carotid artery (instead of the innominate artery) is the first branch originating from the aortic arch. This is followed by left common carotid artery and left subclavian artery. The aberrant right subclavian artery is the last arch branch and originates from the descending thoracic aorta traversing the mediastinum from left to right, behind the trachea and esophagus. An aortic diverticulum can develop in 60% of these cases at the origin of right subclavian artery from the descending thoracic aorta, which appears like a diverticulum, called Kommerell's diverticulum. This can undergo aneurysmal degeneration and rupture.

Right-sided arch occurs in 0.1% of the population and it is associated with an aberrant left subclavian artery in approximately 50% of cases. Various arch branching patterns have been described in these patients. In individuals with a right-sided arch and an aberrant left subclavian artery, the sequence of branches originating from the arch consists of left common carotid artery first, followed by the right common carotid and right subclavian arteries and then the aberrant left subclavian artery. Kommerell's diverticulum can also develop at the origin of right subclavian artery from the descending thoracic aorta. In general, the diverticula of Kommerell and aberrant subclavian arteries can be complicated by aneurysms.

Although the surgical management of arch anomalies is beyond the scope of this review, the surgical cannulation strategies need to be tailored according to the individual anatomy. For the total arch replacement in these patients, a side arm graft can be anastomosed to one of the common carotid arteries for the cardiopulmonary bypass and ACP and additional directed cerebral perfusion can be provided using a balloon-tipped catheter through the other carotid artery, if necessary.

FUTURE APPROACHES

Despite the tremendous improvement in the strategies of end-organ protection and surgical procedures resulting into better surgical outcomes, operative mortality and stroke have remained the major challenges after aortic arch replacement. Exploring the alternate strategies for the aortic arch replacement has recently been a focus of dynamic investigation and innovation. Hybrid and total endovascular approaches for the aortic arch replacement have been devised to provide a less invasive alternates for high-risk patients. For the endovascular procedures aortic arch has been divided into 5 anatomic zones as classified by Ishimaru and colleagues and Criado and colleagues (**Fig. 8**).

HYBRID ARCH REPAIR

Hybrid approaches combine a conventional open arch repair with endovascular techniques. These

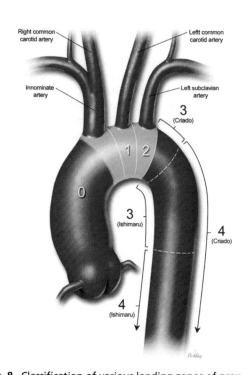

Fig. 8. Classification of various landing zones of proximal aorta for the endovascular arch repair. The aortic arch is the segment that includes the origin of 3 supraaortic branch vessels: the innominate artery, left common carotid artery and left subclavian artery. Two landing zone classifications system, Criado and Ishimaru, are used to describe the proximal aortic anatomy for the purpose of endovascular aortic repair. The landmarks for the proximal aorta are similar in both systems. Zone 0 comprises the ascending aorta and the origin of the innominate artery. Zone 1 involves the origin of left common carotid artery. Zone 2 includes the origin of left subclavian artery. However, both systems differ in their description of the distal aortic landing zones. In the Criado system, zone 3 comprises a short segment of the aorta, which is 2 cm distal to the origin of left subclavian artery, and zone 4 commences where zone 3 ends. In the Ishimaru system, zone 3 is lengthier, spanning from the distal to the origin of left subclavian artery to an imaginary border at the end of the curvature of aortic arch. Zone 4 begins from there on. (*Courtesy of* Baylor College of Medicine, Houston, TX; with permission.)

were developed with the goal to provide a safe and effective surgical alternative to the patients who are either high risk or unfit for a traditional open arch replacement. The goal of hybrid repair is to simplify a multicomponent open surgical repair into an open repair for the debranching of the aortic arch vessels by creating extra-anatomic bypasses. This is followed by a staged or unstaged endovascular procedure to repair the diseased arch and descending thoracic aorta.

Single, double, or total great vessel transposition is performed, followed by thoracic endovascular aortic repair (TEVAR).

The literature on the hybrid aortic arch repair encompasses a wide variety of procedures ranging from TEVAR with left subclavian artery coverage (combined with or without left carotid to subclavian bypass) to zone 0 endovascular repair with double or total arch vessels debranching followed by a TEVAR. Hybrid arch repair also includes patients with extensive thoracic aortic disease involving aortic arch and descending thoracic aorta (**Fig. 9**). Basically, a common element that classifies an arch procedure as a hybrid arch repair is the fact that both open and endovascular techniques are used to repair the entire arch. An individualized approach is adopted for each patient, based on patient's anatomy, comorbidities and surgeon's preference. Plichta and colleagues[35] have proposed a classifications scheme of hybrid arch repair focused on the intensity of mechanical circulatory support needed to perform the repair. Each procedure is further divided into single or dual staged procedure. Of note, a simpler arch debranching procedure using coverage of left subclavian artery combined with the TEVAR was not included in the classification.[35]

Type I Hybrid Arch Repairs

Type I hybrid arch repairs are performed by median sternotomy and using a side-biting clamp on the

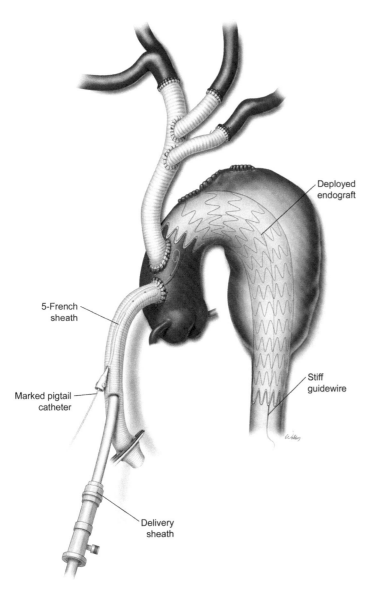

Fig. 9. Depiction of Zone 0 hybrid arch endovascular repair: This procedure is an alternative in select patients with limited arch disease. The aortic arch vessels are debranched and bypasses are created in a double Y-graft fashion. Various configurations can be adopted to debranch the arch branch vessels. A separate graft is used as a conduit for antegrade endovascular deployment of the stent graft. (*Courtesy of* Baylor College of Medicine, Houston, TX; with permission.)

Deployed endograft

5-French sheath

Marked pigtail catheter

Stiff guidewire

Delivery sheath

ascending aorta to perform the debranching of supraaortic vessels. This can be accomplished on a beating heart with or without cardiopulmonary bypass support. This creates a landing zone in the ascending aorta for subsequent TEVAR via an antegrade or retrograde approach.

Type II Hybrid Arch Repairs

Type II hybrid arch repairs are performed using cardiopulmonary bypass support, but without hypothermic circulatory arrest. The heart is stopped to replace the ascending aorta with a surgical graft combined with the debranching of supraaortic vessels. The endograft can be landing into the replaced ascending aorta as a stable landing zone in either antegrade or retrograde fashion as a single or dual staged procedure.

Type III Hybrid Arch Repairs

Type III hybrid arch repairs are performed using cardiopulmonary bypass support with hypothermic circulatory arrest. These repairs are usually performed on the patients who have inadequate landing zone even after debranching of supraaortic vessels mainly owing to extensive multisegment aortic disease. These repairs include the replacement of both the ascending aorta and transverse arch using a standard surgical graft along with creation of an elephant trunk. The elephant trunk can be created using a surgical classic elephant trunk graft or a stent graft also called a frozen elephant trunk. Furthermore, the completion elephant trunk procedure can be performed endovascular as a dual staged repair. Frozen elephant trunk technique is one of the more commonly performed hybrid aortic arch repair procedures.

Postoperative mortality for the hybrid procedure has been reported to be between 6% and 10%, which is comparable with traditional open arch repair, despite the fact that patients with multiple comorbidities are treated with this approach.[35–37] The reported technical success with these procedures has been up to 86%, with the type I endoleak being the most common mode of failure (9%) and 5% to 10% incidence of perioperative stroke.[36,37]

As with any novel surgical technique, once more experience has accumulated with the hybrid arch repairs, new postoperative complications such as spinal cord ischemia, retrograde dissection, stent migration, and endoleaks bring value to the success of these procedures. Moreover, to evaluate the long-term durability and survival of hybrid procedures, their outcomes need to be compared with those of contemporary series of open surgical arch repairs. Despite the usefulness and effectiveness of the hybrid repair, sometimes the open component of hybrid procedure is not suitable or technically feasible for patients with significant comorbidities or unfavorable anatomy. Consequently, total endovascular repair of the aortic arch has emerged as a potential treatment option.

TOTAL ENDOVASCULAR AORTIC REPAIR

With the evolution of endovascular technology new approaches have emerged to repair the aortic arch. Chimney repair and inner-branched endografts are new options to treat aortic arch aneurysms in high-risk patients.

Chimney Repair

In the chimney or parallel graft technique, multiple fenestrated or standard stent grafts are deployed in the arch such that blood will be routed through the main body of the aortic stent graft and through the branched or connection stents. With this technique, the multiple stent grafts are deployed at the same landing site in a way that the chimney graft into the arch vessels is essentially sandwiched between the aortic wall and the main body stent graft. The blood is directed through both the main body aortic graft and the chimney graft, allowing the simultaneous perfusion through the aorta and the arch vessels.

This technique was developed to provide an off-the-shelf endovascular solution to the surgeons, particularly for the patients with emergent aortic pathology where custom-made stent grafts are not an option.[38,39] A standard, commercially available thoracic endograft and any covered or uncovered peripheral vascular stent can be used to perform this procedure.

Some of the limitations inherent to this technique include endoleak, stent migration, and device kinking. In addition, secondary interventions are usually challenging with this approach. The reported perioperative type I endoleak rate with this technique has been 15% to 40%. The incidence of chimney graft occlusion is as high as 11%. Also, there is a considerable rate of stroke both in the perioperative period and upon short-term follow-up.[38] With the unknown long-term durability of this technique combined with the fact that each component of the chimney repair is used off label, this approach is advocated to be reserved as an endovascular bailout option for high-risk symptomatic or ruptured aneurysms.

Custom-Made Scalloped, Fenestrated Devices

Devices have been developed where a scallop at the proximal end of the stent graft provides the perfusion to a single arch single branch vessel such as left subclavian or left common carotid artery. This provides an opportunity to obtain a more proximal seal and expand the landing zone for the limited arch endovascular repair. Small series have described the procedural success using this concept, but large cohort data with this technique are almost nonexistent. Some of the concerns with this technique include type I endoleaks and the technically challenging nature of the procedure needing precise deployment not to cover the intended arch branch vessels.

Arch Branched Endografts

Chuter and colleagues[40] initially reported the use of a modular branched stent graft for the total arch endovascular repair. With this system, double arch extra-anatomic bypasses including carotid–carotid and left common carotid to left subclavian artery bypasses are performed first. Next, a branched stent graft is deployed through the right common carotid approach such that the proximal portion of the graft land in the ascending aorta; a long branch extends in the brachiocephalic/innominate artery and a short, large branch remaining open to the aortic arch. To complete the repair, the next modular component is then delivered through the femoral arterial access, connecting the distal end of the large branch of the Chuter branched device to the descending thoracic aorta.

Although this group has demonstrated the technical success using their device, this approach is limited by technically challenging nature of the procedure needing both carotid and femoral access routes and extreme precision in deployment of the proximal component. Furthermore, delivering the arch device through the carotid artery using a very large delivery sheath (22- to 24-Fr) remains a concern for the adverse neurologic events. This size requirement also limits the number of patients eligible for this device owing to small carotid vessels.[40]

Inner-branched arch endograft

Currently, a third-generation inner-branched endograft (Cook Medical, Bloomington, IN), is available under the investigational device exemption at selected centers. Based on the experience obtained from previous total endovascular arch repair strategies, this device was developed to overcome these challenges.

This new generation, inner-branched device is designed such that its proximal landing zone is in the ascending aorta where either 1 or 2 sealing stents, supported by an active fixation with barbs on the most proximal stent, provides the seal.

Furthermore, to obtain a durable proximal seal, a healthy nondilated proximal aorta, spanning from the sinotubular junction to the innominate artery, is needed for a proximal landing zone.

The graft contains 2 internal branches for connection to the innominate and left common carotid artery. The left subclavian artery is covered and perfused by a left carotid to subclavian bypass or transposition. The graft conforms to the curvature of the arch to achieve a proximal seal, thus minimizing the bird-beaking that is particularly important in gothic arches. The 2 distal stents of branched device provide the distal seal, but more frequently, a distal extension stent graft is needed to completely isolate the aneurysm. A custom iliac limb (Cook Medical) is used as innominate bridging stent. A commercially available covered stent, either a self-expanding Viabahn (Gore, Flagstaff, AZ) or balloon expandable such as Advanta V12 (Atrium, Hudson, NH), can be used to connect the second inner branch to the left common carotid artery. Three-vessel access is required for device deployment. The femoral access is used for the main body graft deployment; left axillary artery provides access for the left common carotid artery covered bridging stent and either the right axillary or right common carotid artery is used for the bridging limb to the innominate artery (**Fig. 10**). Rapid ventricular pacing is used to control the cardiac output for the device deployment.[41,42]

The initial clinical experience with this device was reported in 2012.[42] Successful cannulation of 11 of the 12 branches was achieved in 6 patients. One patient experienced stroke owing to the branch vessels thrombosis and there was 1 endoleak.

Subsequently, Haulon and colleagues[41] published a multicenter report reviewing the initial global experience with this device in 2014. Of note, 6 of the 38 patients in this series were from the initial experience reported earlier. All the patients were significantly high risk or unfit for the open surgical repair. The reported technical success was 84.2%, in 32 of 38 patients. Five patients died within 30 days of the index procedure (13.2%) and there were 6 cerebrovascular complications (4 transient ischemic attacks, 1 stroke, and 1 subarachnoid hemorrhage). The authors noted a higher mortality in first 10 cases (30%) compared with the last 28 patients (7.1%) treated with this technique. Also, the composite risk of early mortality and neurologic complications was significantly higher in the first 10 patients ($P = .019$). In addition, a larger ascending aortic diameter of greater than 38 mm was a significant risks factor for the composite events ($P = .026$). This report emphasized

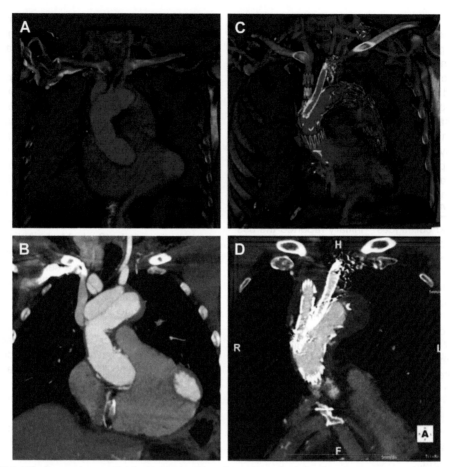

Fig. 10. Total Endovascular aortic Arch repair using Inner-Branched Device: Preoperative (*A, B*) and post-operative (*C, D*) computed angiographic scan images with 3-dimensional volume rendering in a patient with post-dissection aortic arch aneurysm after a previous open type I aortic dissection repair.

that, with proper operator training and patient selection, aortic arch repair is a feasible and safe option for the patients who are not the candidates for conventional open surgical repair.[41]

Recently, 3 high-volume endovascular centers published their combined experience with inner-branched devices after their initial learning curve. They reported significantly improved subsequent outcomes with this technology compared with the initial global experience. They had a 100% procedural success in all 27 patients and no 30-day mortality. Major stroke occurred in 2 patients (7.4%), minor stroke in 1 (3.7%), and 2 patients experienced transient spinal cord ischemia with full recovery (7.4%). There were 3 type II endoleaks and 1 late death from distal aortic rupture. With these favorable outcomes, the authors concluded that this technology should be considered for high-risk patients who are not candidates for traditional open repair.

Another subset of patients who can potentially benefit from this technology is the ones who

develop postdissection aortic arch aneurysm after a previous open type A aortic dissection repair. Previous ascending aortic graft provides a stable landing zone for this technology, making future endovascular arch repair an attractive option to the reoperative sternotomy in high-risk patients. This method is particularly relevant, because aneurysmal degeneration after prior type I aortic dissection constitutes more than one-half of the patients with arch aneurysm. Milne and colleagues[43] recently evaluated the postoperative CT images of 73 patients who underwent acute type A aortic dissection repair at their institution with the goal to assess their anatomic suitability for future arch aneurysm repair using an inner-branched endograft. The noted that almost 70% of patients were anatomically suitable candidates for future arch repair using arch inner-branched endograft. The reasons of exclusion were short ascending aortic surgical graft, graft kinking, or too large of surgical graft diameter. As the arch endovascular repair technology continues to evolve, these anatomic criteria should be considered while fashioning the surgical graft at the time of index aortic dissection operation, for a future arch endovascular repair.

Aftab and colleagues[44] have described their technique of distal arch and descending thoracic aortic repair with frozen elephant trunk in acute type I aortic dissection. In this technique, the stent graft is suture secured into the distal arch as part of the distal aortic anastomosis. The left subclavian artery is covered and a custom-made fenestration is created into the graft to perfuse the artery. The authors reported excellent distal aortic remodeling with expansion of true lumen and obliteration of false lumen in the stented aorta. A theoretic advantage of using the frozen elephant trunk technique in patient undergoing acute type I dissection repair is that it can provide a stable proximal and distal landing zone for future total arch endovascular repair in case of arch aneurysmal degeneration. This might be particularly helpful for the patients who are significantly high risks to undergo a reoperative sternotomy and total arch repair.

Although these initial reports have established the technical feasibility of total endovascular arch repair, this technology is still in its early stages. As the current technology is evolving there are quite a few challenges ahead. These arch endografts are available only at a few centers of excellence. There is a steep learning curve related to this technology. Additionally, patients with ascending aortic diameter greater than 38 cm are not suitable candidates for this therapy and there is a need for low-prolife devices to minimize access site complications, as the internal diameter of current delivery system is 22- to 24-Fr. Finally, the long-term durability of this technology is uncertain and will need to be evaluated.

SUMMARY

There has been tremendous improvement in the field of aortic arch surgery in the last 2 decades. A better understanding of the effects of brain and systemic ischemia during circulatory arrest, refinements in techniques of brain and end-organ protection, and liberal use of ACP and moderate hypothermia have made arch repair safer. Likewise, surgical approaches such as traditional/ frozen elephant trunk, trifurcated graft, 4-branch graft, and skirted graft have truly revolutionized the field of arch surgery. As endovascular technology and open surgical techniques are evolving, aortic surgeons will continue to learn and incorporate these in their routine practice, with the goal to provide the best outcomes to our patients.

ACKNOWLEDGMENTS

The authors thank Joseph S. Coselli, MD and Baylor College of Medicine for the permission to reproduce their illustrations, Scott A. Weldon, MA, CMI, for creating the medical illustrations, and Hajra F. Khan, BS, JD, for contributing to the editing of the article.

REFERENCES

1. Svensjo S, Bengtsson H, Bergqvist D. Thoracic and thoracoabdominal aortic aneurysm and dissection: an investigation based on autopsy. Br J Surg 1996; 83:68–71.
2. Brenner DJ, Hall EJ. Computed tomography–an increasing source of radiation exposure. N Engl J Med 2007;357:2277–84.
3. Cascade PN, Leibel SA. Decision-making in radiotherapy for the cancer patient: the American College of Radiology appropriateness criteria project. CA Cancer J Clin 1998;48:146–50.
4. Parker MS, Matheson TL, Rao AV, et al. Making the transition: the role of helical CT in the evaluation of potentially acute thoracic aortic injuries. AJR Am J Roentgenol 2001;176:1267–72.
5. Shellock FG, Spinazzi A. MRI safety update 2008: part 1, MRI contrast agents and nephrogenic systemic fibrosis. AJR Am J Roentgenol 2008;191:1129–39.
6. Cayne NS, Veith FJ, Lipsitz EC, et al. Variability of maximal aortic aneurysm diameter measurements on CT scan: significance and methods to minimize. J Vasc Surg 2004;39:811–5.
7. Singh K, Jacobsen BK, Solberg S, et al. Intra- and interobserver variability in the measurements of abdominal aortic and common iliac artery diameter with computed tomography. The Tromso study. Eur J Vasc Endovasc Surg 2003;25:399–407.
8. Bonnafy T, Lacroix P, Desormais I, et al. Reliability of the measurement of the abdominal aortic diameter by novice operators using a pocket-sized ultrasound system. Arch Cardiovasc Dis 2013;106:644–50.
9. Elefteriades JA, Farkas EA. Thoracic aortic aneurysm clinically pertinent controversies and uncertainties. J Am Coll Cardiol 2010;55:841–57.
10. Bischoff MS, Brenner RM, Scheumann J, et al. Long-term outcome after aortic arch replacement with a trifurcated graft. J Thorac Cardiovasc Surg 2010; 140:S71–6 [discussion: S86–91].
11. Di Bartolomeo R, Berretta P, Pantaleo A, et al. Long-term outcomes of open arch repair after a prior aortic operation: our experience in 154 patients. Ann Thorac Surg 2017;103(5):1406–12.
12. Moulakakis KG, Mylonas SN, Markatis F, et al. A systematic review and meta-analysis of hybrid aortic arch replacement. Ann Cardiothorac Surg 2013;2:247–60.

13. Tian DH, Croce B, Hardikar A. Aortic arch surgery. Ann Cardiothorac Surg 2013;2:245.

14. Hiratzka LF, Bakris GL, Beckman JA, et al, American College of Cardiology Foundation, American Heart Association Task Force on Practice Guidelines, American Association for Thoracic Surgery, American College of Radiology, American Stroke Association, Society of Cardiovascular Anesthesiologists, Society for Cardiovascular Angiography and Interventions, Society of Interventional Radiology, Society of Thoracic Surgeons, Society for Vascular Medicine. 2010 ACCF/AHA/AATS/ACR/ASA/SCA/SCAI/SIR/STS/SVM guidelines for the diagnosis and management of patients with thoracic aortic disease: a report of the American College of Cardiology Foundation/American Heart Association Task Force on practice guidelines, American Association for Thoracic Surgery, American College of Radiology, American Stroke Association, Society of Cardiovascular Anesthesiologists, Society for Cardiovascular Angiography and Interventions, Society of Interventional Radiology, Society of Thoracic Surgeons, and Society for Vascular Medicine. Circulation 2010;121:e266–369.

15. Erbel R, Aboyans V, Boileau C, et al, Guidelines ESCCfP. 2014 ESC Guidelines on the diagnosis and treatment of aortic diseases: document covering acute and chronic aortic diseases of the thoracic and abdominal aorta of the adult. The Task Force for the Diagnosis and Treatment of Aortic Diseases of the European Society of Cardiology (ESC). Eur Heart J 2014;35:2873–926.

16. Bigelow WG, Callaghan JC, Hopps JA. General hypothermia for experimental intracardiac surgery; the use of electrophrenic respirations, an artificial pacemaker for cardiac standstill and radio-frequency rewarming in general hypothermia. Ann Surg 1950;132:531–9.

17. Barcroft H, Samaan A. The explanation of the increase in systemic flow caused by occluding the descending thoracic aorta. J Physiol 1935;85:47–61.

18. Gross RE. Treatment of certain aortic coarctations by homologous grafts; a report of nineteen cases. Ann Surg 1951;134:753–68.

19. Cooley DA, De Bakey ME. Surgical considerations of intrathoracic aneurysms of the aorta and great vessels. Ann Surg 1952;135:660–80.

20. Debakey ME. Successful resection of aneurysm of distal aortic arch and replacement by graft. J Am Med Assoc 1954;14:1398–403.

21. Creech O Jr, Debakey ME, Mahaffey DE. Total resection of the aortic arch. Surgery 1956;40:817–30.

22. Borst HG, Schaudig A, Rudolph W. Arteriovenous fistula of the aortic arch: repair during deep hypothermia and circulatory arrest. J Thorac Cardiovasc Surg 1964;48:443–7.

23. Griepp RB, Stinson EB, Hollingsworth JF, et al. Prosthetic replacement of the aortic arch. J Thorac Cardiovasc Surg 1975;70:1051–63.

24. Guilmet D, Roux PM, Bachet J, et al. A new technic of cerebral protection. Surgery of the aortic arch. Presse Med 1986;15:1096–8 [in French].

25. Spielvogel D, Strauch JT, Minanov OP, et al. Aortic arch replacement using a trifurcated graft and selective cerebral antegrade perfusion. Ann Thorac Surg 2002;74:S1810–4 [discussion: S1825–32].

26. Kazui T, Washiyama N, Muhammad BA, et al. Total arch replacement using aortic arch branched grafts with the aid of antegrade selective cerebral perfusion. Ann Thorac Surg 2000;70:3–8 [discussion: 8–9].

27. Kouchoukos NT, Wareing TH, Murphy SF, et al. Sixteen-year experience with aortic root replacement. Results of 172 operations. Ann Surg 1991;214:308–18 [discussion: 318–20].

28. Borst HG, Walterbusch G, Schaps D. Extensive aortic replacement using "elephant trunk" prosthesis. Thorac Cardiovasc Surg 1983;31:37–40.

29. Carrel T, Althaus U. Extension of the "elephant trunk" technique in complex aortic pathology: the "bidirectional" option. Ann Thorac Surg 1997;63:1755–8.

30. Carrel T, Berdat P, Kipfer B, et al. The reversed and bidirectional elephant trunk technique in the treatment of complex aortic aneurysms. J Thorac Cardiovasc Surg 2001;122:587–91.

31. Kato M, Ohnishi K, Kaneko M, et al. New graft-implanting method for thoracic aortic aneurysm or dissection with a stented graft. Circulation 1996;94:II188–93.

32. Ma WG, Zhu JM, Zheng J, et al. Sun's procedure for complex aortic arch repair: total arch replacement using a tetrafurcate graft with stented elephant trunk implantation. Ann Cardiothorac Surg 2013;2:642–8.

33. Martens A, Beckmann E, Kaufeld T, et al. Total aortic arch repair: risk factor analysis and follow-up in 199 patients. Eur J Cardiothorac Surg 2016;50:940–8.

34. Preventza O, Bakaeen FG, Stephens EH, et al. Innominate artery cannulation: an alternative to femoral or axillary cannulation for arterial inflow in proximal aortic surgery. J Thorac Cardiovasc Surg 2013;145:S191–6.

35. Plichta RP, Aftab M, Roselli EE. Current management of aortic arch lesions with hybrid procedures: a tailored approach to a progressive disease. J Cardiovasc Surg (Torino) 2016;57:437–47.

36. Czerny M, Weigang E, Sodeck G, et al. Targeting landing zone 0 by total arch rerouting and TEVAR: midterm results of a transcontinental registry. Ann Thorac Surg 2012;94:84–9.

37. Preventza O, Aftab M, Coselli JS. Hybrid techniques for complex aortic arch surgery. Tex Heart Inst J 2013;40:568–71.

38. Mangialardi N, Serrao E, Kasemi H, et al. Chimney technique for aortic arch pathologies: an 11-year single-center experience. J Endovasc Ther 2014; 21:312–23.

39. Wilson A, Zhou S, Bachoo P, et al. Systematic review of chimney and periscope grafts for endovascular aneurysm repair. Br J Surg 2013;100:1557–64.

40. Chuter TA, Schneider DB, Reilly LM, et al. Modular branched stent graft for endovascular repair of aortic arch aneurysm and dissection. J Vasc Surg 2003;38:859–63.

41. Haulon S, Greenberg RK, Spear R, et al. Global experience with an inner branched arch endograft. J Thorac Cardiovasc Surg 2014;148:1709–16.

42. Lioupis C, Corriveau MM, MacKenzie KS, et al. Treatment of aortic arch aneurysms with a modular transfemoral multibranched stent graft: initial experience. Eur J Vasc Endovasc Surg 2012;43: 525–32.

43. Milne CP, Amako M, Spear R, et al. Inner-branched endografts for the treatment of aortic arch aneurysms after open ascending aortic replacement for type a dissection. Ann Thorac Surg 2016;102: 2028–35.

44. Aftab M, Plichta R, Roselli E. Acute Debakey type I dissection repair using frozen elephant trunk: the Cleveland Clinic technique. Semin Cardiothorac Vasc Anesth.

Type B Aortic Dissections
Current Guidelines for Treatment

Daniel B. Alfson, MD, Sung W. Ham, MD*

KEYWORDS

- Stanford type B aortic dissection • False lumen • Treatment • TEVAR • Remodeling

KEY POINTS

- Stanford type B aortic dissections (TBADs) involve the descending aorta and are further classified by time of onset and presence of complications.
- Diagnosis begins with clinical suspicion and is confirmed with imaging of the entire aorta.
- Anti-impulse medical therapy is the cornerstone of treatment and should be initiated immediately on diagnosis for all aortic dissections.
- Thoracic endovascular aortic repair (TEVAR) is indicated in patients with complicated TBAD as well as during the subacute phase in high-risk patients with uncomplicated TBAD.
- Surveillance imaging with serial CT angiography (CTA) is mandatory to identify potential disease progression and device-related complications.

INTRODUCTION
Pathophysiology

Aortic dissections are a subclass of acute aortic pathology characterized by a tear in the innermost layer of the aortic wall, the intima, allowing some of the blood flow to escape from the main passageway (the true lumen [TL]) of the aorta and reroute into an artificial secondary passageway (the false lumen [FL]) between the intima and media of the aortic wall. This entry tear can be located anywhere along the length of the aorta (**Fig. 1**). Driven by the high pressure within the aorta, the flow of blood through the entry tear leads to separation of the layers of the aortic wall and subsequent propagation of the FL either antegrade or retrograde along the aorta or occasionally in both directions. This constellation of events can disrupt normal blood flow resulting in clinically significant malperfusion to vital organs or weakening of the aortic wall with ensuing aortic rupture.[1,2]

Classification and Prognosis

Aortic dissections are classified based on the anatomic distribution of the dissection, the time from symptom onset, and the presence of complications. Using these classifications, clinicians gain significant prognostic information that aid in developing the most effective treatment plan individualized for each patient.

Anatomic distribution

The aorta is divided into distinct anatomic segments. The ascending aorta and the aortic arch are the first 2 segments, encompassing the portion of the aorta from its root up to and including the left subclavian artery (LSCA), and the descending aorta begins just distal to the LSCA and includes the thoracic and abdominal portions of the aorta. In 1965, DeBakey and colleagues[3] used these anatomic segments to classify aortic dissections into 3 separate types according to anatomic involvement: type I involves both the ascending

Disclosure Statement: The authors have nothing to disclose.
Division of Vascular Surgery, Department of Surgery, Keck School of Medicine of USC, University of Southern California, 1520 San Pablo Street, HCC II, Suite 4300, Los Angeles, CA 90033-5330, USA
* Corresponding author.
E-mail address: Sung.Ham@med.usc.edu

Cardiol Clin 35 (2017) 387–410
http://dx.doi.org/10.1016/j.ccl.2017.03.007
0733-8651/17/© 2017 Elsevier Inc. All rights reserved.

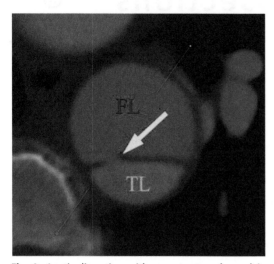

Fig. 1. Aortic dissection with an entry tear (*arrow*) in an intimal flap separating the TL from the FL, as seen on axial view of CTA. (*From* Tolenaar JL, van Keulen JW, Trimarchi S, et al. Number of entry tears is associated with aortic growth in type B dissections. Ann Thorac Surg 2013;96(1):40; with permission.)

distribution of dissections directly affects patient outcomes. Mortality was significantly improved when patients with aortic dissections involving the ascending aorta received surgical versus medical treatment, whereas this treatment effect was not seen in those having dissections involving only the descending aorta. This finding, therefore, led to the development of the more widely used Stanford classification: type A aortic dissections involve the ascending aorta or the aortic arch, whereas TBADs involve only the descending aorta (**Fig. 2**).

This notion that anatomic distribution of aortic dissections has significant prognostic implications has been supported in numerous subsequent studies.[5–8] One such report examined patient data from the International Registry of Acute Aortic Dissection (IRAD), a large consortium currently comprising 30 referral centers in 11 countries that was established in 1996 to evaluate the current management and outcomes of aortic dissections.[9] Using an early version of this database, Hagan and colleagues[10] reviewed approximately 500 cases of aortic dissections demonstrating results similar to those in Daily and colleagues'[4] article from 3 decades earlier. Patients with type A dissections who underwent surgical repair had lower mortality (26%) than those treated medically (58%), whereas the mortality of those with type B dissections was lower when treated medically (11%) than with surgery (31%). Furthermore, these

and descending aorta, type II is isolated to the ascending aorta and the aortic arch, and type III is isolated to the descending aorta (further subdivided into IIIa and IIIb).

Shortly thereafter, Daily and colleagues[4] at Stanford University discovered that anatomic

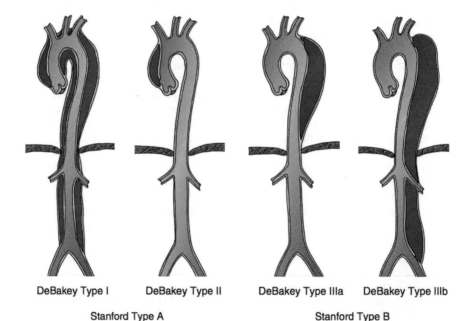

DeBakey Type I   DeBakey Type II   DeBakey Type IIIa   DeBakey Type IIIb

Stanford Type A   Stanford Type B

Fig. 2. Classification of aortic dissections by anatomic distribution using the DeBakey and Stanford systems. (*From* Conrad MF, Cambria RP. Aortic dissection. In: Cronenwett JL, Johnston KW, editors. Rutherford's vascular surgery. 8th edition. Philadelphia: Saunders, Elsevier Inc; 2014. p. 2170.e4; with permission.)

results are validated in a more recent IRAD study demonstrating lower cumulative survival in patients with type A aortic dissections versus TBADs[11] (**Fig. 3**).

The anatomic distribution of aortic dissections thus plays a significant prognostic role in directing management. Type A aortic dissections represent surgical emergencies and are managed by resecting and replacing the ascending aortic segment containing the proximal entry tear. On the contrary, TBADs traditionally have been treated medically, with surgical intervention reserved only for complicated presentations with malperfusion syndrome or rupture. With technological advancements in thoracic endografts, the role of TEVAR in the treatment of TBAD is currently in evolution. A growing body of evidence supporting the use of TEVAR in the treatment of TBAD has led to a paradigm shift in how this challenging disease is approached. To further examine these exciting developments, the remainder of the discussion focuses on TBADs.

Time of onset

Although there remains some disparity regarding its delineation into clinically relevant time frames, time of symptom onset also serves as a useful method for classifying TBAD. The classification system on which many influential studies and even current management guidelines have been structured[10,12–14] is based on an early autopsy series defining acute dissections as those diagnosed within 14 days of symptom onset and chronic dissections as those diagnosed beyond 14 days, because the majority were diagnosed postmortem within 14 days.[15] The disparity with this classification arose with the advent of modern diagnostic modalities and treatment strategies because current survival trends have changed significantly. In 2013, Booher and colleagues[11] described an updated classification based on IRAD data. After stratifying patients with TBAD according to management type, individual inflection points according to time interval from symptom onset were identified, defining 4 distinct time periods: hyperacute (within 24 hours), acute (2–7 days), subacute (8–30 days), and chronic (>30 days). Survival continued to decrease for up to 30 days after symptom onset, after which it plateaued into the chronic phase, demonstrating that acute presentations of TBAD are more aggressive than chronic (**Fig. 4**). These results establish the prognostic significance of using a temporal classification.

Presence of complications

TBAD can be further described as complicated or uncomplicated depending on the presence or absence, respectively, of 1 or more direct clinical

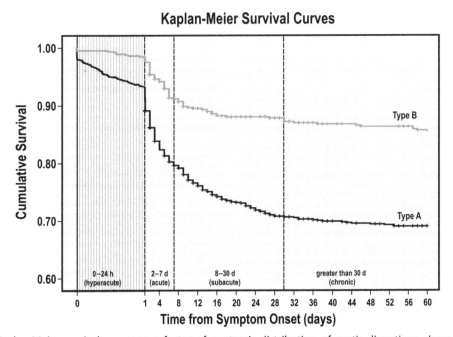

Fig. 3. Kaplan-Meier survival curves as a factor of anatomic distribution of aortic dissections, demonstrating lower short-term cumulative survival with type A compared with type B dissections. (*From* Booher AM, Isselbacher EM, Nienaber CA, et al. The IRAD classification system for characterizing survival after aortic dissection. Am J Med 2013;126(8):730.e22; with permission.)

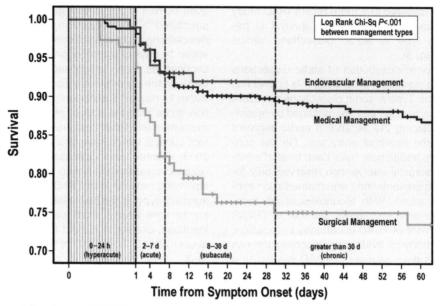

Fig. 4. Survival of patients with TBAD per treatment type demonstrates a clear association with time from symptom onset, as divided into 4 phases according to distinct inflection points: hyperacute, acute, subacute, and chronic. (*From* Booher AM, Isselbacher EM, Nienaber CA, et al. The IRAD classification system for characterizing survival after aortic dissection. Am J Med 2013;126(8):730.e22; with permission.)

consequences of the dissection. Complicated TBAD is defined by the presence of at least one of the following: malperfusion syndrome (visceral or lower extremity), aortic rupture, hypotension or shock, neurologic sequelae, recurrent or refractory pain, hypertension refractory to medical therapy, early aortic dilation, or propagation of the dissection.[1] Those remaining cases of TBAD without these signs and symptoms on presentation and during the hospital course are considered uncomplicated.

Approximately 25% to 40% of TBAD cases are complicated, with approximately 10% of these secondary to malperfusion.[14,16] Malperfusion occurs when there is end-organ ischemia secondary to obstruction of 1 or more visceral aortic branches and/or the lower extremities. Two variations are described in the literature: dynamic and static malperfusion[17,18] (**Fig. 5**). Dynamic malperfusion is responsible for approximately 80% of all cases of malperfusion and is caused by a mobile intimal flap that intermittently obstructs the artery orifice with each ventricular beat as the increased flow in the FL compresses the TL. Static obstruction occurs when the dissection extends directly into the branches, causing luminal narrowing and possibly formation of a distal thrombus. This type of obstruction is unlikely to resolve with restoration of aortic TL flow alone and may require endovascular stenting.[19]

Patients with complicated TBAD have worse in-hospital survival (50%) compared with those with uncomplicated (90%).[1] Long-term outcomes are similarly distinct, as demonstrated by a single-center retrospective review of patients presenting with acute TBAD over a 13-year period[16] (**Fig. 6**). This concept is further supported by an IRAD study that demonstrated TBAD patients with branch vessel involvement were approximately 3 times more likely to die, and those with hypotension/shock were approximately 24 times more likely to die.[20]

DISSECT classification

In light of the contemporary advancements in endovascular treatment options, particularly for TBAD, a new succinct classification system was developed.[21] This mnemonic-based classification system is called DISSECT, which includes 6 characteristics that are important when choosing the best contemporary management option for TBAD, many of which are previously discussed. The temporal classification in this system is based the 14-day acute phase (**Box 1**).

EPIDEMIOLOGY AND RISK FACTORS

The yearly incidence of aortic dissections as a group historically has been reported as 3 to 4 per 100,000 persons[22,23]; however, a more recent review of more than 30,000 patients

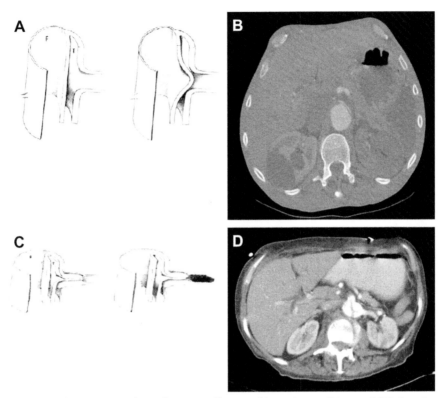

Fig. 5. Types of malperfusion in complicated TBAD as illustrated by artist rendition and CTA imaging: (*A, B*) dynamic malperfusion and (*C, D*) static malperfusion. (*From* Parsa CJ, Hughes GC. Surgical options to contend with thoracic aortic pathology. Semin Roentgenol 2009;44(1):34; with permission.)

in Sweden reported a much higher yearly incidence of 15 per 100,000 persons.[24] TBAD accounts for approximately 25% to 40% of all aortic dissections,[25,26] with a yearly incidence of approximately 2 per 100,000 persons.[27] An IRAD review of 4428 patients with aortic dissections over a 17-year period demonstrated 33% having TBAD, the average age of which was 64 years, and two-thirds were men.[28]

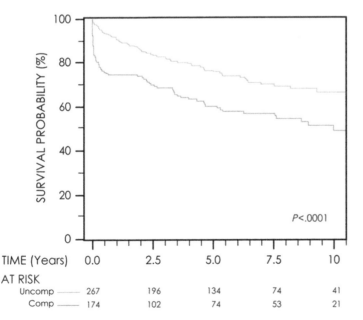

Fig. 6. Long-term survival of patients with complicated (Comp) TBAD is lower than those with uncomplicated (Uncomp) TBAD. (*From* Afifi RO, Sandhu HK, Leake SS, et al. Outcomes of patients with acute type B (DeBakey III) aortic dissection: a 13-year, single-center experience. Circulation 2015;132(8):752; with permission.)

TIME (Years)	0.0	2.5	5.0	7.5	10
AT RISK					
Uncomp	267	196	134	74	41
Comp	174	102	74	53	21

P<.0001

Box 1
The DISSECT system of classifying aortic dissections

D, Duration

  Ac = acute: less than 2 weeks from initial onset of symptoms

  Sa = subacute: 2 weeks to 3 months after symptom onset

  Ch = chronic: greater than 3 months from initial symptom onset

I, Intimal

  Tear, A = ascending aorta

  Ar = aortic arch

  D = descending aorta

  Ab = abdominal aorta

  Un = unknown

S, size of aorta

Maximum center-line diameter in millimeters

SE, segmental extent of involvement

A = ascending aorta exclusively

  Ar = aortic arch exclusively

  D = descending exclusively

  Ab = abdomen exclusively

  AAr = ascending to arch

  AD = ascending to descending

  AAb = ascending to abdomen

  AI = ascending to iliac

  ArD = arch to descending

  ArAb = arch to abdomen

  ArI = arch to iliac

  DAb = descending to abdomen

  DI = descending to iliac

C, clinical complications

  C = complicated

    Aortic valve involvement

    Cardiac tamponade

    Rupture

    Branch vessel malperfusion

    Progression of aortic involvement

    Other – uncontrollable hypertension or symptoms, rapid FL dilation,

    and/or transaortic diameter enlargement greater than 10 mm within 2 weeks

  UC = uncomplicated

T, thrombosis of FL

  P = patent aortic FL

  CT = complete thrombosis of FL

    A = ascending aorta

    Ar = aortic arch

D = descending aorta

Ab = abdominal aorta

PT = partial thrombosis of FL

A = ascending aorta

Ar = aortic arch

D = descending aorta

Ab = abdominal aorta

From Dake MD, Thompson M, van Sambeek M, et al. DISSECT: a new mnemonic-based approach to the categorization of aortic dissection. Eur J Vasc Endovasc Surg 2013;46(2):175–90; with permission.

Risk factors for TBAD include a wide variety of conditions that either place excess stress on the aortic wall or decrease its strength.[29] Excess aortic wall stress occurs secondary to uncontrolled arterial hypertension, smoking, hyperlipidemia, atherosclerosis, cocaine or stimulant use, pregnancy, deceleration trauma, or iatrogenic injury. Moreover, the most commonly identified risk factor for TBAD is arterial hypertension, which is found in up to 80% of cases in some reports.[10] Conditions that decrease the strength of the aortic wall include genetic connective tissue disorders, such as Marfan syndrome, Ehlers-Danlos syndrome, and Loeys -Dietz syndrome, as well as inflammatory vasculitides, such as Takayasu arteritis, giant cell arteritis, and Behçet's Disease.

DIAGNOSIS
Clinical History and Physical Examination

The diagnosis of TBAD is primarily clinical with confirmation based on imaging studies.[30] The most common presenting complaint is severe or worst-ever pain typically described as sharp (68%) rather than tearing or ripping (52%).[10] Most (89%) patients describe this pain as occurring abruptly, located most often in the back (64%–70%), chest (63%–67%), or abdomen (43%), with few patients (20%–25%) describing migratory pain.[10,20,28,29,31] Patients may also present with other signs or symptoms indicating the presence of complications, such as syncope, stroke, decreased consciousness, spinal cord ischemia with neurologic deficits, mesenteric ischemia with abdominal pain, acute renal failure, or lower extremity ischemia.[30]

On physical examination, most (60%–70%) are hypertensive and few (2%–3%) are hypotensive or in shock. Approximately 10% to 20% have pulse deficits, with few patients (2%–3%) having signs of ischemia to the central or peripheral nervous system.[10,20,28]

Laboratory Testing

Laboratory tests are of limited usefulness in securing the diagnosis of TBAD, but they can be helpful adjuncts in the assessment of possible complications and their severity. Most tests are aimed at evaluating the presence and extent of end-organ ischemia, such as renal failure or bowel ischemia. Patients presenting with signs or symptoms of TBAD should undergo laboratory testing, including complete blood cell count, troponin, arterial blood gas, creatinine kinase, creatinine, liver function tests, and lactate. An elevated D dimer specifically within the first hour of presentation has been found to increase the diagnostic suspicion for TBAD.[31,32]

Diagnostic Imaging

Physicians must have a low clinical threshold for pursuing diagnostic imaging as a means for securing the diagnosis.[1] Historically, diagnostic imaging was limited to the chest radiograph in search of an abnormal aortic contour, with aortography as the confirmatory test.[33] With the advent and improvement of modern imaging modalities, however, such as CTA, MRI, and transesophageal echocardiography (TEE), diagnostic sensitivity has increased significantly.

CTA is the gold standard for the diagnosis of TBAD due to its wide availability, high resolution, and speed of image acquisition. Both the sensitivity and specificity of CTA of the chest, abdomen, and pelvis in identifying aortic dissections approach 100%, with the presence of an intimal flap separating 2 lumens as the key diagnostic finding. Alternative imaging modalities that have similarly acceptable diagnostic accuracy include MRI and TEE. Although TEE has a lower diagnostic sensitivity (80%) than both CTA and MRI, it is the second-line imaging modality after CTA because it is faster, portable, and more readily available than MRI.[32,34]

Not only does imaging serve to secure the diagnosis of TBAD but also it aids in choosing the most fitting treatment option because no case of TBAD is anatomically identical. In addition to establishing the diagnosis, the role of imaging in TBAD is to comprehensively assess the entire aorta and its branches to both delineate the extent of dissection and identify key pathologic features that are key to directing treatment.

TREATMENT
Historical Perspectives

Aortic dissections were originally described by Morgagni in 1761. Meaningful treatment of this rapidly lethal condition was initially limited because antemortem diagnosis was infrequent. Moreover, until the invention of cardiopulmonary bypass in the mid-1950s, surgical management was essentially impossible.[10] The first report of successful open surgical repair of aortic dissections was published in 1955 by DeBakey and colleagues,[35] awakening hope, albeit short-lived, for an effective treatment option for this lethal condition. In subsequent years, however, during which open repair was performed, unfavorably high rates of morbidity and mortality were seen, with paraplegia occurring in 30% to 36% of patients and mortality rates of up to 50%.[1] Consequently, open surgical repair soon fell out of favor, leading to the first of 2 major paradigm shifts in the management of TBAD.

In 1965, Wheat and colleagues[36] demonstrated the first successful management of TBAD using medical treatment alone, reporting 100% survival of 4 patients with TBAD treated with aggressive blood pressure control. This idea was subsequently supported by the influential report by Daily and colleagues[4] in 1970, which established the Stanford classification system. The results of these studies, as well as other subsequent studies,[37,38] are responsible for the paradigm shift in the management of TBAD from surgical intervention to medical treatment aimed at reducing blood pressure and heart rate. Medical management remained the standard of care for patients with TBAD over the next few decades until, in the mid-1990s, significant advancements were made in the development and application of endovascular technology, giving rise to another shift in the management paradigm.

Endovascular therapy for aortic dissections was introduced in 1994 with the first report of successful TEVAR by Dake and colleagues[39] This report, as well as a subsequent report by Dake and colleagues[40] in 1999, served as the basis for introducing the concept of using endograft technology as a safe and effective treatment option for TBAD, especially because initial success rates were encouragingly high: 93% to 100% for acute TBAD and 78% to 100% for chronic TBAD.[1] This concept was further expanded by a prospective study in 1999 by Nienaber and colleagues,[41] which demonstrated that TEVAR was a better therapeutic option for complicated TBAD compared with traditional open surgical repair. In a matched comparison of 12 patients who underwent TEVAR versus 12 who underwent open repair, TEVAR resulted in no morbidity or mortality, but open repair resulted in 33% mortality and 42% morbidity within 12 months.

Soon thereafter, commercial medical product developers began producing and refining their own versions of endografts for the treatment of aortic dissections. The first endograft approved by the US Food and Drug Administration (FDA) for the treatment of TBAD was the Gore TAG Thoracic Endoprosthesis (W. L. Gore and Associates, Flagstaff, AZ) in late 2013, followed soon thereafter by the Valiant Thoracic Stent Graft with Captivia Delivery System (Medtronic, Minneapolis, MN) in early 2014. Currently, there are 3 FDA-approved endografts for the treatment of TBAD. Although TEVAR continues to show promise as an effective treatment option, medical therapy has remained the cornerstone of the initial treatment of TBAD.

Medical Treatment

The first-line treatment of acute TBAD is medical therapy, appropriately termed, *anti-impulse therapy*, aimed at minimizing the changes in pressure that the aortic wall experiences over time.[42] All patients with TBAD should be treated with anti-impulse therapy immediately on diagnosis.[19] Subsequently, medical treatment strategies may be subdivided into acute or chronic therapy.

Acute medical treatment
Successful anti-impulse therapy is accomplished by aggressively controlling blood pressure and heart rate. Control of blood pressure is intuitively important for patients with aortic dissections, with a widely accepted goal systolic pressure of 100 mm Hg to 120 mm Hg.[29] Less intuitive but also important is control of heart rate, as demonstrated in a study by Kodama and colleagues.[43] In this study, patients were treated with a variety of antihypertensive medications to maintain appropriate systolic blood pressure. Those patients with average heart rates of less than 60 beats per minute (bpm) during their initial hospitalization had much better long-term outcomes than those with heart rates of greater than or equal to 60 bpm in terms of freedom from aortic events and freedom from surgical intervention (**Fig. 7**).

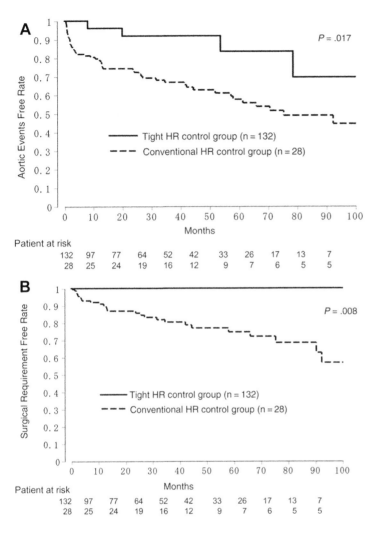

Fig. 7. Tighter heart rate control in patients with acute TBAD is associated with greater (A), freedom from aortic events, and (B), surgical requirement, specifically in those with heart rates less than 60 bpm. (*From* Kodama K, Nishigami K, Sakamoto T, et al. Tight heart rate control reduces secondary adverse events in patients with type B acute aortic dissection. Circulation 2008;118(14 Suppl):S169–70; with permission.)

Intravenous (IV) β-adrenergic receptor blockers are most frequently used as the first-line treatment of aortic dissections, with IV calcium channel blockers (CCBs) a commonly favored alternative option.[1] Recent data have demonstrated a significant survival difference between the 2 classes of medications compared between treatment of type A versus type B dissections. Suzuki and colleagues[44] found that the use of CCB was associated with improved overall survival selectively in those with type B versus type A dissections, whereas the use of β-adrenergic receptor blockers was not (**Fig. 8**). For refractory hypertension, IV angiotensin-converting enzyme inhibitors and vasodilators should be considered.[1]

Those few patients who present with hypotension or shock should receive rapid volume expansion with the judicious addition of IV vasopressors. Although it is tempting to aim for normal

physiologic blood pressures, permissive hypotension should be the therapeutic goal to avoid progression of the dissection and/or rupture. Pain control is also critically important and should not be overlooked. If any of these clinical manifestations is persistent or refractory to aggressive medical management, consideration for disease progression should be given and appropriate intervention should be promptly undertaken.[1]

Chronic medical treatment

In those patients with uncomplicated acute TBAD who achieve successful acute medical treatment with blood pressure and heart rate control, transition of IV to oral chronic antihypertensive therapy is a widely accepted treatment option,[29,31,45,46] with the long-term goal of preventing aortic expansion and favoring aortic remodeling, as discussed later.[1] This is often termed, *optimal medical therapy* [*OMT*]. The choice of antihypertensive

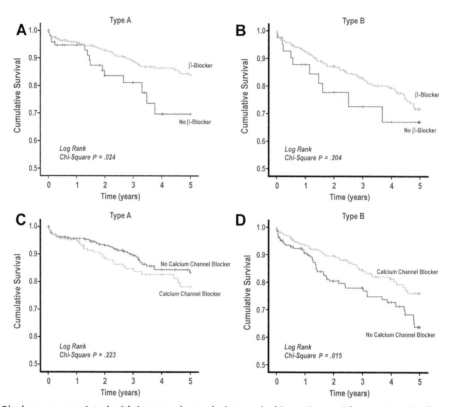

Fig. 8. β-Blockers are associated with improved cumulative survival in patients with type A aortic dissections but not TBADs (*A, B*), whereas the opposite association is seen in CCBs (*C, D*). (*From* Suzuki T, Isselbacher EM, Nienaber CA, et al. Type-selective benefits of medications in treatment of acute aortic dissection (from the International Registry of Acute Aortic Dissection [IRAD]). Am J Cardiol 2012;109(1):125; with permission.)

medication for use in chronic TBAD is still a matter of debate and deserves additional long-term prospective studies; however, current data suggest best outcomes occur with CCB and, if coronary artery disease is also present, a statin.[47] Several studies have validated the effectiveness of CCB as part of the regimen for OMT in TBAD, with long-term results demonstrating decreased aortic expansion[48] and increased survival.[49]

Most patients require multiple antihypertensive medications to achieve OMT. One small series of patients with chronic aortic dissections reported a median of 4 antihypertensive medications per patient was necessary to achieve a 60% success rate of effective blood pressure control (defined as <135/80 mm Hg). Those patients in whom medical therapy failed were younger and more obese.[50]

Endovascular Repair (Thoracic Endovascular Aortic Repair)

In general, the primary goal of TEVAR is to cover the primary entry tear with an endograft, thereby expanding the TL and restoring normal blood flow. The resultant depressurization of the FL prevents progression of the dissection, with the eventual goal of inducing FL thrombosis and protective aortic remodeling[51,52] (**Fig. 9**). With the preponderance of recent data supporting the use of endovascular repair of TBAD, all patients should be considered for TEVAR, even those patients with uncomplicated TBAD who have been successfully treated with acute medical therapy alone. It remains helpful, however, to distinguish between complicated and uncomplicated TBAD while determining the best treatment option.

Complicated type B aortic dissections

Patients diagnosed with complicated acute TBAD should receive emergent TEVAR after the initiation of anti-impulse medical therapy. This recommendation is supported by a wealth of published data comparing TEVAR to OMT, traditional open surgical repair, or both. Dialetto and colleagues[53] found TEVAR superior to OMT alone in patients with complicated TBAD. In 2008, Szeto and colleagues[54] validated the results of the earlier Nienaber and colleagues'[41] study, demonstrating significantly better outcomes in terms of mortality

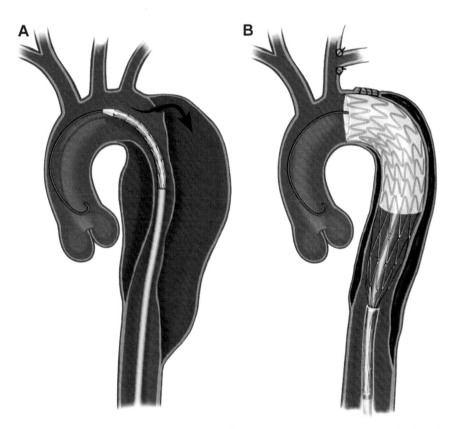

Fig. 9. (*A*) TBAD with an undeployed endograft positioned over the proximal entry tear just distal to the LSCA. (*B*) The deployed endograft covers the proximal entry tear with the goal of inducing FL thrombosis and TL re-expansion. A transposition of the LSCA to the left common carotid artery is illustrated. (*From* Conrad MF, Cambria RP. Aortic dissection. In: Cronenwett JL, Johnston KW, editors. Rutherford's vascular surgery. 8th edition. Philadelphia: 2014. p. 2179.e4; with permission.)

and morbidity compared with open surgical repair. This study retrospectively analyzed 35 patients with acute TBAD complicated by either rupture (51.4%) or malperfusion (48.6%) over a 4-year period. Technical success was 97.1% with 30-day mortality of only 2.8%, significantly lower than that of open surgical repair (29.3%). Another single-institution retrospective study from the University of Pennsylvania[55] analyzed the outcomes of 77 patients with acute complicated TBAD after either TEVAR, open surgical repair, or OMT; 30-day mortality was significantly lower in the TEVAR group (4%) compared with either the open surgical repair group (40%) or OMT group (33%). Long-term outcomes were similarly impressive with significantly improved survival at 1 year, 3 years, and 5 years in those who underwent TEVAR (82%, 79%, and 79%, respectively). Several meta-analyses reporting short-term and midterm results of patients with complicated TBAD repaired with TEVER also support these findings.[56–58] Taken together, these results have led

to the widely publicized recommendation that TEVAR is the gold standard for acute complicated TBAD.[26,29,31,46]

Uncomplicated type B aortic dissections

Stable patients who present with uncomplicated TBAD have historically been treated with OMT alone because short-term outcomes comparing OMT with TEVAR were initially promising.[45,59] Long-term results from IRAD, however, comparing medically treated uncomplicated TBAD patients with those treated with TEVAR favor the latter, with 1 study demonstrating 29% mortality in the medical group compared with 16% in the TEVAR group at a follow-up interval of 5 years[60] (**Fig. 10**). More recently, Durham and colleagues[61] published their experience at Massachusetts General Hospital with acute, uncomplicated TBAD, reporting that although long-term intervention-free survival of medically managed TBAD was similar to those treated with TEVAR, more than 40% eventually required repair. Furthermore, the

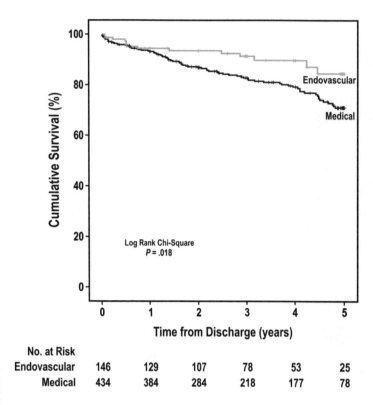

Fig. 10. Long-term cumulative survival of patients with uncomplicated TBAD is improved after endovascular intervention compared with medical treatment alone. (*From* Fattori R, Montgomery D, Lovato L, et al. Survival after endovascular therapy in patients with type B aortic dissection: a report from the International Registry of Acute Aortic Dissection (IRAD). JACC Cardiovasc Interv 2013;6(8):879; with permission.)

medically treated group had failed medical therapy in 58% with 38% mortality and 29% eventually undergoing aortic-related interventions. More interesting is the inflection point on the survival curve that occurs at the 2-year mark whereby the subgroup who underwent intervention in the first place had better survival than those who did not at the end of the follow-up period (**Fig. 11**). The results

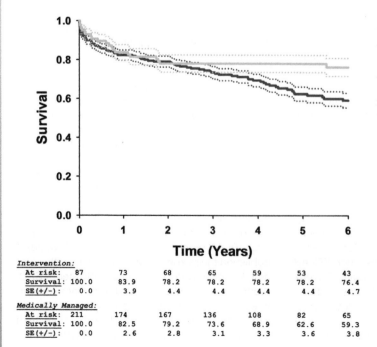

Fig. 11. Long-term survival of patient with uncomplicated TBAD who were treated with TEVAR is better than those who were treated medically, with an inflection point seen at 2 years reflecting divergence of survival between the 2 groups. SE, standard error. (*From* Durham CA, Cambria RP, Wang LJ, et al. The natural history of medically managed acute type B aortic dissection. J Vasc Surg 2015;61(5):1197; with permission.)

of these studies have ignited interest in the beneficial role of TEVAR in patients with uncomplicated TBAD. Few randomized controlled trials have been conducted to assess the clinical benefit of elective TEVAR in these patients,[1] 1 of which was the INSTEAD trial.

The INSTEAD (INvestigation of STEnt Grafts in Aortic Dissection) trial included 140 patients with uncomplicated TBAD in the subacute and chronic phases and compared OMT alone with OMT and TEVAR. Initial 2-year data published in 2009 failed to demonstrate a significant survival difference between OMT and TEVAR + OMT.[12] The INSTEAD-XL study, however, provided extended follow-up of 5 years and revealed the mortality curve diverged between years 2 and 5, with TEVAR having lower aorta-specific mortality (7% vs 19%) and trending toward lower overall mortality (11% vs 19%) compared with the OMT group[62] (**Fig. 12**). Both short-term and long-term data from this trial also demonstrated that TEVAR had a significantly greater effect on what is referred to as aortic remodeling. Findings of the INSTEAD-XL trial underscore the importance of long-term surveillance in patients with TBAD and that the benefit of TEVAR materializes over late follow-up.

Aortic Remodeling

The term, *aortic remodeling*, is used to describe a series of favorable morphologic changes that occur in the aorta after placement of an aortic endograft, such as expansion of the TL, regression of the FL, stabilization of the transaortic diameter, and complete thrombosis of the FL. The concept of monitoring these distinct morphologic changes after TEVAR was first suggested in 2006 by Eggebrecht and colleagues[57] and was subsequently proved of clinical importance by the INSTEAD-XL trial as well as numerous other morphologic studies.[63–67] These results suggest that OMT alone may only serve to delay aortic aneurysmal degeneration because significant aortic aneurysm formation has been found to occur in up to 25% to 30% of these patients within 4 years.[68] This idea that gradual, long-term changes in aortic morphology after endograft placement are protective serves as the premise of the unfolding recommendation that TEVAR should be considered a beneficial treatment option for patients with uncomplicated TBAD. This raises the questions of which patients with uncomplicated TBAD should undergo repair and how they can be identified at initial presentation.

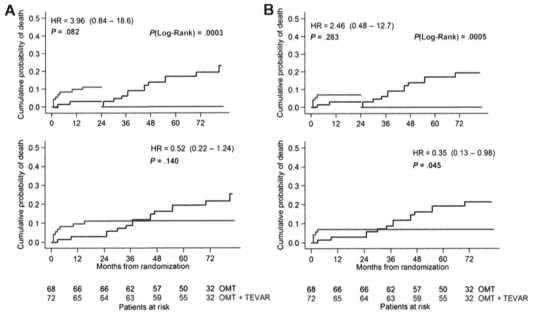

Fig. 12. Long-term results of the INSTEAD-XL trial. (*A*) All-cause mortality was lower in patients who received both OMT + TEVAR compared with OMT alone, although this was only a trend. (*B*) Aortic-specific mortality was significantly lower in patients who received both OMT + TEVAR compared with OMT alone. HR, hazard ratio. (*From* Nienaber CA, Kische S, Rousseau H, et al. Endovascular repair of type B aortic dissection: long-term results of the randomized investigation of stent grafts in aortic dissection trial. Circ Cardiovasc Interv 2013;6(4):412; with permission.)

High-Risk Features

Several predictive anatomic features of both acutely and chronically dissected aorta have been identified that serve to characterize certain patients with uncomplicated TBAD as high risk for the development of aneurysmal degeneration and who, therefore, would derive the most benefit from TEVAR[68]:

Aortic diameter greater than 40 mm: although some conflicting results appear in the literature,[48] an aortic diameter greater than 40 mm at initial presentation has been identified as a predictor of aortic growth by several reports.[69–74] Additionally, IRAD data have shown an increased likelihood of complications and greater in-hospital mortality of TBAD patients who present initially with aortic diameters greater than or equal to 55 mm.[75]

Patent false lumen with partial thrombosis: the presence of a patent FL alone is a predictor of aortic growth and poor outcomes,[70–72,74,76,77] whereas complete thrombosis of the FL is associated with intuitively better outcomes.[70,72,78] Furthermore, Tsai and colleagues[79] demonstrated that partial thrombosis of the FL is associated with poor outcomes. The mechanism behind this is thought to be due to the hemodynamic impact of the partial thrombosis, where the pressure inside the FL is increased due to obliteration of distal outflow (**Fig. 13**). This hypothesis has recently been supported in animal models.[80]

False lumen diameter greater than or equal to 22 mm: results of Song and colleagues[81] demonstrated that an FL diameter of greater than or equal to 22 mm, when measured at the upper descending thoracic aorta, was associated with late aneurysm formation as well as higher event rates, including those related to the aneurysm and death.

Single proximal entry tear, greater than or equal to 10 mm in size: patients with 1 entry tear at presentation exhibit higher aortic growth rate than those who have multiple entry tears.[82] Larger tears that are more proximal to the LSCA have similarly undesirable outcomes.[83]

Elliptical true lumen with saccular false lumen: this configuration is associated with increased aortic growth, with an odds ratio of approximately 5.0, as demonstrated in 1 study[84] (**Fig. 14**).

Rapid aortic enlargement greater than 4 mm per year: this is a recommendation from an international consensus document on the management of TBAD.[14]

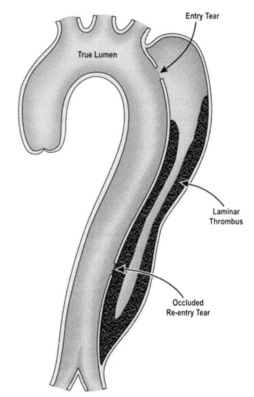

Fig. 13. Type B aortic dissection with patent entry tear, partial thrombosis of the false lumen, and obliteration of the distal outflow, leading to increased false lumen pressure. (*From* Tsai TT, Schlicht MS, Khanafer K, et al. Tear size and location impacts false lumen pressure in an ex vivo model of chronic type B aortic dissection. J Vasc Surg 2008;47(4):844–851; with permission.)

Chronic aneurysm diameter greater than or equal to 55 mm: aortic diameters greater than 55 mm to 60 mm have an estimated 30% yearly risk of rupture.[29]

Recurrent and/or refractory pain and refractory hypertension: these clinical signs are independent predictors of in-hospital mortality, and ensuing endovascular intervention is associated with improved outcome compared with medical management alone.[85]

Timing

The main question that remains unanswered in the treatment of patients with uncomplicated but high-risk TBAD, therefore, is when to perform the TEVAR. At present, there are no high-quality data comparing timing of interventions in uncomplicated TBAD. INSTEAD-XL excluded acute dissections by design, with a median time to intervention of 57 days.[62] The only available data on timing

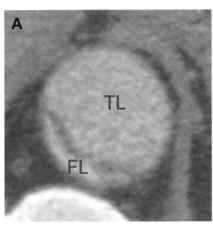 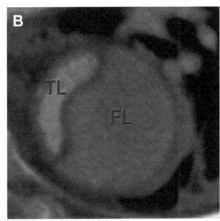

Fig. 14. Axial CTA imaging demonstrating (*A*) circular TL with compressed FL and (*B*) an elliptical TL with saccular FL. (*From* Tolenaar JL, van Keulen JW, Jonker FHW, et al. Morphologic predictors of aortic dilatation in type B aortic dissection. J Vasc Surg 2013;58(5):1222; with permission.)

comes from studies of patients with complicated TBAD. One such study used the Virtue registry[86] to examine outcomes of 100 patients who were treated with the Medtronic Valiant endograft over a 3-year period. Patients were divided into 3 groups: acute (<15 days), subacute (15–92 days), and chronic (>92 days). The acute phase group had lower dissection-related survival compared with chronic and subacute groups. Favorable aortic remodeling, however, as measured by FL thrombosis, was seen in both acute and subacute groups, where chronic had greater persistent FL flow (**Fig. 15**). These results suggest that TEVAR be performed in the subacute phase (14–90 days) because it is during this phase that better outcomes overlap, in terms of survival and favorable aortic remodeling.

Another relevant study that had timing data is STABLE.[65] In this prospective, multicenter study, patients with complicated TBAD were repaired using a PETTICOAT (Provisional ExTension To Induce COmplete ATtachment) concept with a stent graft proximally and uncovered stent distally, both produced by Cook Medical (Bloomington, IN) (**Fig. 16**). Patients were divided into an acute group (≤14 days) and a nonacute group (>14 days). In the midterm, overall results were excellent with 89.3% freedom from aorta-related events at 2 years, and 43.5% complete thrombosis of the FL in the thoracic aorta. Results at 2 years from both the acute and nonacute groups demonstrated expansion of the thoracic TL and regression of the FL. Continued expansion of the abdominal FL, however, was seen in the acute group, whereas regression occurred in the nonacute group.

Together, the results of these studies can be extrapolated to suggest that TEVAR should be performed during the subacute phase in patients with uncomplicated, high-risk TBAD, because those performed in the acute phase have a higher complication rates. Furthermore, aortic plasticity, or capacity for favorable aortic remodeling, seems preserved through subacute phase.

Technical Considerations

After making the determination that TEVAR is indicated as treatment of TBAD, extensive but meticulous preprocedure planning is critical to maximize its therapeutic efficacy while minimizing the risk of procedure-related complications. With the growing number of available aortic endografts (currently there are 3 commercially available devices produced by Gore, Medtronic, and Cook), each with its own pros and cons, choosing the correct device for implantation is an important part of this planning. This decision is typically based on a combination of patient-specific aortic and access vessel anatomy, device characteristics, surgeon preference, and device availability. Regarding spinal cord protection, preoperative insertion of a cerebral spinal fluid drainage catheter is routine for all elective TEVAR procedures. For emergent TEVAR, lumbar drains are placed postoperatively as needed if patients develop paraplegia.[87,88]

In the operating room, routine use of intravascular ultrasound[89–91] and/or TEE[92,93] facilitates wire access and confirmation in the TL, as well as aiding in proper stent sizing and identifying potential immediate intraoperative complications (**Fig. 17**). Achieving a proximal seal is critical to prevent persistent antegrade pressurization of the FL and the complications that may subsequently ensue.[1] This is accomplished both by

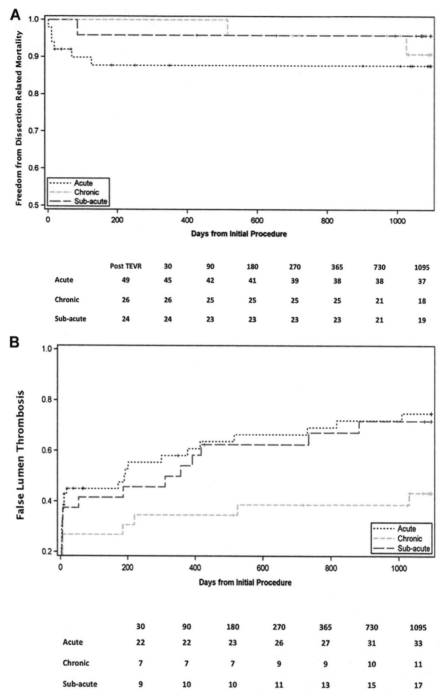

Fig. 15. VIRTUE Registry results showing (A), lower dissection-related survival in acute TBAD patients compared with subacute and chronic, and (B), greater FL thrombosis in both acute and subacute TBAD patients compared with chronic. (*From* VIRTUE Registry Investigators. Mid-term outcomes and aortic remodeling after thoracic endovascular repair for acute, subacute, and chronic aortic dissection: the VIRTUE Registry. Eur J Vasc Endovasc Surg 2014;48(4):363–71; with permission.)

oversizing the endograft up to 10% of the aortic diameter proximal to the dissected segment in normal aorta[94,95] as well as having a proximal aortic neck length, or landing zone, of at least 2 cm.[96,97] Not infrequently, the LSCA requires coverage to achieve a proximal seal. In emergent TEVAR, the LSCA is routinely covered if required and revascularized later if indicated. An exception

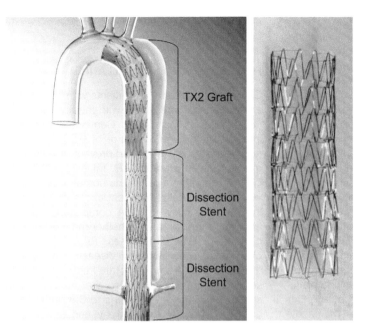

Fig. 16. The PETTICOAT endograft design. (*From* Lombardi JV, Cambria RP, Nienaber CA, et al. Prospective multicenter clinical trial (STABLE) on the endovascular treatment of complicated type B aortic dissection using a composite device design. J Vasc Surg 2012;55(3):632.e2; with permission.)

to this is a patient with an existing left internal mammary artery to coronary artery bypass; in this case, a left common carotid to LSCA bypass with LSCA embolization would be carried out at the same setting of TEVAR. For all elective TEVAR for TBAD, the authors preferentially transpose the LSCA to the left common carotid artery. Otherwise, the LSCA is bypassed if the patient has a left internal mammary artery coronary bypass graft.[98] After deployment, post–balloon dilation is avoided due to the risk of retrograde type A dissection or aortic rupture.[99–101] Furthermore, if 2 or more endografts are required, the authors avoid building up from distal to proximal because the distal device may cover the exit fenestration

and lead to full pressurization of the FL from the proximal entry tear, thereby increasing the risk of aortic rupture.

After coverage of the proximal entry tear, further intervention depends on the initial indication for treatment. In the case of uncomplicated TBAD, a completion aortogram demonstrating the absence of contrast flow in the FL to the level of the endograft, together with complete patency of downstream visceral branch vessels, is an acceptable endpoint with plan to reassess with CT imaging. On the contrary, when malperfusion is the initial indication, extension of the aortic endograft distally to the celiac artery or selective branch vessel stenting may be necessary if downstream

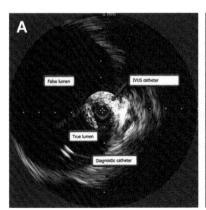
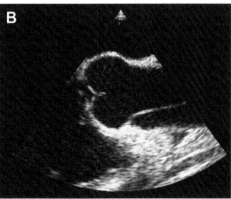

Fig. 17. Adjunct equipment helpful in the operating room when performing TEVAR includes (*A*) intravascular ultrasound (IVUS) and (*B*) TEE. (*From* Hughes GC, Andersen ND, McCann RL. Management of acute type B aortic dissection. J Thorac Cardiovasc Surg 2013;145(3 Suppl):S205; with permission.)

flow remains inadequate. The decision to stent branches is typically based on the clinical, rather than radiologic, severity of malperfusion. The topic of extent of aortic coverage and branch vessel management at the initial time of TEVAR is an issue of controversy and no consensus currently exists. The authors' approach to the initial TEVAR for acute TBAD, whether uncomplicated or complicated, is to cover the primary entry tear with a short endograft with selective distal extension and reassessment with CT imaging in correlation with the clinical status of the patient.

In cases of TBAD complicated by rupture or aneurysm, complete thrombosis of the FL is essential to save a patient's life. This may necessitate extension of the TEVAR down to the celiac artery together with one of several adjunctive procedures aimed at occluding the FL. Various FL treatment procedures are used in the chronic setting and include placement of double-barrel Amplatzer vascular plugs (St. Jude Medical, St. Paul, MN),[102,103] the candy-plug technique,[104,105] and the Knickerbocker technique[106] (**Fig. 18**). A recent study has demonstrated that FL procedures like these are both safe and successful in promoting complete FL thrombosis in the long term when used in patients with TBAD involving the abdominal aorta.[107]

Open Surgical Repair

Because of the significant advancements in endovascular technology, open surgical repair of TBAD has become increasingly rare and is reserved only for a select group of patients. Compared with TEVAR, the morbidity and mortality of open repair of TBAD remain prohibitively high[26,108–110]; hence, it is generally indicated for patients who have already failed or are not amenable to TEVAR. Patients with genetic connective tissue disorders, such as Marfan, Ehlers-Danlos, and Loeys-Dietz syndromes, represent a unique group of patients given the fragility of their tissues and uncertain long-term durability of endografts in this disease group. Open repair remains, however, the procedure of choice in this patient population.[29,31]

Open repair is usually performed via a left anterolateral thoracotomy, with or without cardiopulmonary bypass. The aortic segment containing the intimal tear is resected and replaced with a prosthetic graft. In cases of TBAD that are complicated by visceral malperfusion, extension of this resection and replacement can be performed to include affected visceral branches. Alternatively, surgical fenestration can be performed, which involves widely resecting the dissected septum via an aortotomy to relieve branch obstruction and equalize flow between the true and FLs. Extra-

anatomic bypass is considered if lower extremity ischemia is present.[1,30]

FOLLOW-UP AND SURVEILLANCE

Outpatient monitoring of patients with TBAD after acute management, either with medical or surgical therapy, is mandatory. Continuation of anti-impulse therapy with control of blood pressure and heart rate is essential to prevent disease progression, even after TEVAR. Imaging with serial CTA of the entire aorta is the cornerstone of surveillance. General recommendations include having the first follow-up CTA completed 1 month after acute presentation whether managed medically or with TEVAR to assess for device-related changes or progression of disease. Findings on the 1 month CTA should dictate frequency of subsequent imaging. If stable, the next imaging should be obtained 3 months to 6 months later, and subsequently followed by annual imaging. Any change in clinical presentation (ie, pain, refractory hypertension, or signs of end-organ ischemia) should prompt immediate reimaging, followed by the appropriate intervention if positive.[30]

FUTURE DIRECTIONS

Expertise in aortic dissections, specifically TBADs, is a misnomer because there remains much to be learned about this complex vascular pathology in terms of early diagnosis, risk-prediction, and optimal therapeutic strategies. An array of several biomarkers, such as smooth muscle myosin heavy chain, soluble elastin fragments, polycistin 1, and D dimer, are being analyzed as potential indicators for early diagnosis of acute aortic dissections.[111] Based on in vitro models of hemodynamic flow within dissected aortas,[112] current research examining flow dynamics in aortic dissections using 4-D flow-sensitive MRI technology is providing interesting information on alterations of aortic blood flow patterns in aortic dissections that may be helpful in identifying additional prognostic indicators heralding development of future complications or disease progression.[113] Refinements of aortic endograft technology, including branched and fenestrated endografts, is enabling patient-specific stent placement,[114] this being a response to 1 of several important questions with regard to using TEVAR in the management of TBAD, including how distal to extend the endograft,[115] as well as what happens to the perfusion pattern of the downstream dissected aorta and its branches after TEVAR.[116] These are only a few of the many exciting research topics that are currently being

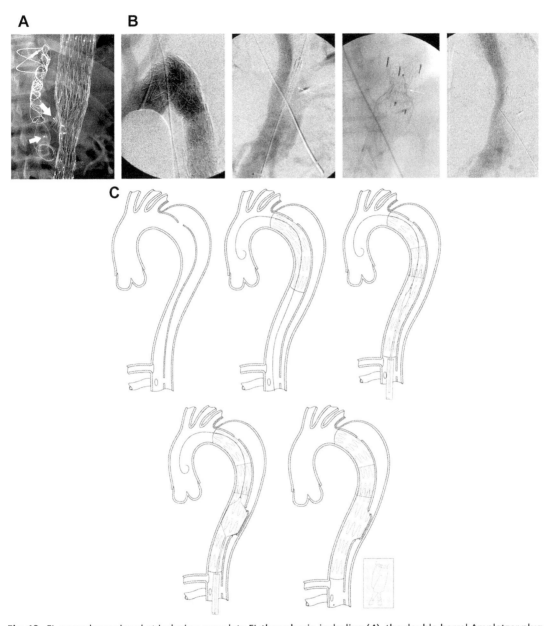

Fig. 18. FL procedures aimed at inducing complete FL thrombosis, including (*A*), the double-barrel Amplatzer plug (*arrows*), (*B*), the candy-plug technique, and (*C*), the Knickerbocker technique. (*From* [*A*] Yong XZE, Nixon I, Brooks M. Aortic intimal defect occlusion with dual AMPLATZER plugs. J Vasc Interv Radiol 2016;27(6):866, with permission; [*B*] Ogawa Y, Nishimaki H, Chiba K, et al. Candy-plug technique using an excluder aortic extender for distal occlusion of a large false lumen aneurysm in chronic aortic dissection. J Endovasc Ther 2016;23(3):483–6, with permission; and [*C*] Kölbel T, Carpenter SW, Lohrenz C, et al. Addressing persistent false lumen flow in chronic aortic dissection: the knickerbocker technique. J Endovasc Ther 2014;21(1):117–22, with permission.)

examined and hold much promise in advancing this field of cardiovascular medicine and surgery.

REFERENCES

1. Nauta FJ, Trimarchi S, Kamman AV, et al. Update in the management of type B aortic dissection. Vasc Med 2016;21(3):251–63.

2. Criado FJ. Aortic dissection: a 250-year perspective. Tex Heart Inst J 2011;38(6):694–700.

3. DeBakey ME, Henly WS, Cooley DA, et al. Surgical management of dissecting aneurysms of the aorta. J Thorac Cardiovasc Surg 1965;49:130–49.

4. Daily PO, Trueblood HW, Stinson EB, et al. Management of acute aortic dissections. Ann Thorac Surg 1970;10(3):237–47.

5. Appelbaum A, Karp RB, Kirklin JW. Ascending vs descending aortic dissections. Ann Surg 1976; 183(3):296–300.

6. Wolfe WG, Moran JF. The evolution of medical and surgical management of acute aortic dissection. Circulation 1977;56(4):503–5.

7. Mills SE, Teja K, Crosby IK, et al. Aortic dissection: surgical and nonsurgical treatments compared. An analysis of seventy-four cases at the University of Virginia. Am J Surg 1979;137(2):240–3.

8. Vecht RJ, Besterman EM, Bromley LL, et al. Acute dissection of the aorta: long-term review and management. Lancet 1980;1(8160):109–11.

9. International Registry of Acute Aortic Dissections. IRAD Website. Available at: http://www.iradonline. org/irad.html. Accessed November 15, 2016.

10. Hagan PG, Nienaber CA, Isselbacher EM, et al. The international registry of acute aortic dissection (IRAD): new insights into an old disease. JAMA 2000;283(7):897–903.

11. Booher AM, Isselbacher EM, Nienaber CA, et al. The IRAD classification system for characterizing survival after aortic dissection. Am J Med 2013; 126(8):730.e19-24.

12. Nienaber CA, Rousseau H, Eggebrecht H, et al. Randomized comparison of strategies for type B aortic dissection: the investigation of STEnt Grafts in Aortic Dissection (INSTEAD) trial. Circulation 2009;120(25):2519–28.

13. Brunkwall J, Lammer J, Verhoeven E, et al. ADSORB: a study on the efficacy of endovascular grafting in uncomplicated acute dissection of the descending aorta. Eur J Vasc Endovasc Surg 2012;44(1):31–6.

14. Fattori R, Cao P, De Rango P, et al. Interdisciplinary expert consensus document on management of type B aortic dissection. J Am Coll Cardiol 2013; 61:1661–78.

15. Hirst AE, Johns VJ, Kime SW. Dissecting aneurysm of the aorta: a review of 505 cases. Medicine (Baltimore) 1958;37(3):217–79.

16. Afifi RO, Sandhu HK, Leake SS, et al. Outcomes of patients with acute type B (DeBakey III) aortic dissection: a 13-year, single-center experience. Circulation 2015;132(8):748–54.

17. Atkins MD, Black JH, Cambria RP. Aortic dissection: perspectives in the era of stent-graft repair. J Vasc Surg 2006;43(Suppl A):30A–43A.

18. Parsa CJ, Hughes GC. Surgical options to contend with thoracic aortic pathology. Semin Roentgenol 2009;44(1):29–51.

19. Scott AJ, Bicknell CD. Contemporary management of acute type B dissection. Eur J Vasc Endovasc Surg 2016;51(3):452–9.

20. Suzuki T, Mehta RH, Ince H, et al. Clinical profiles and outcomes of acute type B aortic dissection in the current era: lessons from the International Registry of Aortic Dissection (IRAD). Circulation 2003;108(Suppl 1):II312–7.

21. Dake MD, Thompson M, van Sambeek M, et al, DEFINE Investigators. DISSECT: a new mnemonic-based approach to the categorization of aortic dissection. Eur J Vasc Endovasc Surg 2013;46(2): 175–90.

22. Mészáros I, Mórocz J, Szlávi J, et al. Epidemiology and clinicopathology of aortic dissection. Chest 2000;117(5):1271–8.

23. Giujusa T, Dario C, Risica G, et al. Aortic dissection: an incidence study based on hospital cases. Cardiologia 1994;39(2):107–12.

24. Landenhed M, Engström G, Gottsäter A, et al. Risk profiles for aortic dissection and ruptured or surgically treated aneurysms: a prospective cohort study. J Am Heart Assoc 2015;4(1):e001513.

25. Hughes GC, Andersen ND, McCann RL. Management of acute type B aortic dissection. J Thorac Cardiovasc Surg 2013;145(3 Suppl):S202–7.

26. Fattori R, Tsai TT, Myrmel T, et al. Complicated acute type B dissection: is surgery still the best option? A report from the International Registry of Acute Aortic Dissection. JACC Cardiovasc Interv 2008;1(4):395–402.

27. Acosta S, Blomstrand D, Gottsäter A. Epidemiology and long-term prognostic factors in acute type B aortic dissection. Ann Vasc Surg 2007; 21(4):415–22.

28. Pape LA, Awais M, Woznicki EM, et al. Presentation, diagnosis, and outcomes of acute aortic dissection: 17-year trends from the international registry of acute aortic dissection. J Am Coll Cardiol 2015;66(4):350–8.

29. Hiratzka LF, Bakris GL, Beckman JA, et al. 2010 ACCF/AHA/AATS/ACR/ASA/SCA/SCAI/SIR/ STS/SVM guidelines for the diagnosis and management of patients with thoracic aortic disease. A report of the American College of Cardiology Foundation/American Heart Association Task Force on Practice Guidelines, American Association for Thoracic Surgery, American College of Radiology, American Stroke Association, Society of Cardiovascular Anesthesiologists, Society for Cardiovascular Angiography and Interventions, Society of Interventional Radiology, Society of Thoracic Surgeons, and Society for Vascular Medicine. J Am Coll Cardiol 2010;55(14):e27–129.

30. Jain V, Farber MA, Vallabhaneni R. Management of acute type B aortic dissections. Expert Rev Cardiovasc Ther 2016;14(9):1043–52.

31. Erbel R, Aboyans V, Boileau C, et al. 2014 ESC Guidelines on the diagnosis and treatment of aortic diseases: document covering acute and chronic aortic diseases of the thoracic and abdominal aorta of the adult. The Task Force for the Diagnosis and Treatment of Aortic Diseases of the European

Society of Cardiology (ESC). Eur Heart J 2014; 35(41):2873–926.

32. Cooper M, Hicks C, Ratchford EV, et al. Diagnosis and treatment of uncomplicated type B aortic dissection. Vasc Med 2016;21(6):547–52.

33. Slater EE, DeSanctis RW. The clinical recognition of dissecting aortic aneurysm. Am J Med 1976;60(5): 625–33.

34. Moore AG, Eagle KA, Bruckman D, et al. Choice of computed tomography, transesophageal echocardiography, magnetic resonance imaging, and aortography in acute aortic dissection: international Registry of Acute Aortic Dissection (IRAD). Am J Cardiol 2002;89(10):1235–8.

35. DeBakey ME, Cooley DA, Creech O. Surgical considerations of dissecting aneurysm of the aorta. Ann Surg 1955;142(4):586–610 [discussion:611–2].

36. Wheat MW, Palmer RF, Bartley TD, et al. Treatment of dissecting aneurysms of the aorta without surgery. J Thorac Cardiovasc Surg 1965;50:364–73.

37. Elefteriades JA, Lovoulos CJ, Coady MA, et al. Management of descending aortic dissection. Ann Thorac Surg 1999;67(6):2002–5 [discussion: 2014–9].

38. Umaña JP, Lai DT, Mitchell RS, et al. Is medical therapy still the optimal treatment strategy for patients with acute type B aortic dissections? J Thorac Cardiovasc Surg 2002;124(5):896–910.

39. Dake MD, Miller DC, Semba CP, et al. Transluminal placement of endovascular stent-grafts for the treatment of descending thoracic aortic aneurysms. N Engl J Med 1994;331(26):1729–34.

40. Dake MD, Kato N, Mitchell RS, et al. Endovascular stent–graft placement for the treatment of acute aortic dissection. N Engl J Med 1999;340(20): 1546–52.

41. Nienaber CA, Fattori R, Lund G, et al. Nonsurgical reconstruction of thoracic aortic dissection by stent-graft placement. N Engl J Med 1999; 340(20):1539–45.

42. Prokop EK, Palmer RF, Wheat MW. Hydrodynamic forces in dissecting aneurysms. In-vitro studies in a Tygon model and in dog aortas. Circ Res 1970; 27(1):121–7.

43. Kodama K, Nishigami K, Sakamoto T, et al. Tight heart rate control reduces secondary adverse events in patients with type B acute aortic dissection. Circulation 2008;118(14 Suppl):S167–70.

44. Suzuki T, Isselbacher EM, Nienaber CA, et al. Type-selective benefits of medications in treatment of acute aortic dissection (from the International Registry of Acute Aortic Dissection [IRAD]). Am J Cardiol 2012;109(1):122–7.

45. Estrera AL, Miller CC, Goodrick J, et al. Update on outcomes of acute type B aortic dissection. The Ann Thorac Surg 2007;83(2):S842–5 [discussion: S846–50].

46. Svensson LG, Kouchoukos NT, Miller DC, et al. Expert consensus document on the treatment of descending thoracic aortic disease using endovascular stent-grafts. Ann Thorac Surg 2008;85: S1–41.

47. Tazaki J, Morimoto T, Sakata R, et al. Impact of statin therapy on patients with coronary heart disease and aortic aneurysm or dissection. J Vasc Surg 2014;60(3):604–12.e2.

48. Jonker FHW, Trimarchi S, Rampoldi V, et al. Aortic expansion after acute type B aortic dissection. The Ann Thorac Surg 2012;94(4):1223–9.

49. Sakakura K, Kubo N, Ako J, et al. Determinants of long-term mortality in patients with type B acute aortic dissection. Am J Hypertens 2009;22(4): 371–7.

50. Eggebrecht H, Schmermund A, Birgelen von C, et al. Resistant hypertension in patients with chronic aortic dissection. J Hum Hypertens 2005; 19(3):227–31.

51. Andacheh ID, Donayre C, Othman F, et al. Patient outcomes and thoracic aortic volume and morphologic changes following thoracic endovascular aortic repair in patients with complicated chronic type B aortic dissection. J Vasc Surg 2012;56(3): 644–50 [discussion: 650].

52. Mani K, Clough RE, Lyons OTA, et al. Predictors of outcome after endovascular repair for chronic type B dissection. Eur J Vasc Endovasc Surg 2012; 43(4):386–91.

53. Dialetto G, Covino FE, Scognamiglio G, et al. Treatment of type B aortic dissection: endoluminal repair or conventional medical therapy? Eur J Cardiothorac Surg 2005;27(5):826–30.

54. Szeto WY, McGarvey M, Pochettino A, et al. Results of a new surgical paradigm: endovascular repair for acute complicated type B aortic dissection. The Ann Thorac Surg 2008;86(1):87–93 [discussion: 93–4].

55. Zeeshan A, Woo EY, Bavaria JE, et al. Thoracic endovascular aortic repair for acute complicated type B aortic dissection: superiority relative to conventional open surgical and medical therapy. J Thorac Cardiovasc Surg 2010;140(6 Suppl): S109–15 [discussion: S142–S146].

56. Luebke T, Brunkwall J. Outcome of patients with open and endovascular repair in acute complicated type B aortic dissection: a systematic review and meta-analysis of case series and comparative studies. J Cardiovasc Surg (Torino) 2010;51(5): 613–32.

57. Eggebrecht H, Nienaber CA, Neuhäuser M, et al. Endovascular stent-graft placement in aortic dissection: a meta-analysis. Eur Heart J 2006; 27(4):489–98.

58. Moulakakis KG, Mylonas SN, Dalainas I, et al. Management of complicated and uncomplicated acute

type B dissection. A systematic review and meta-analysis. Ann Cardiothorac Surg 2014;3(3):234–46.

59. Trimarchi S, Tolenaar JL, Tsai TT, et al. Influence of clinical presentation on the outcome of acute B aortic dissection: evidences from IRAD. J Cardiovasc Surg (Torino) 2012;53(2):161–8.

60. Fattori R, Montgomery D, Lovato L, et al. Survival after endovascular therapy in patients with type B aortic dissection: a report from the International Registry of Acute Aortic Dissection (IRAD). JACC Cardiovasc Interv 2013;6(8):876–82.

61. Durham CA, Cambria RP, Wang LJ, et al. The natural history of medically managed acute type B aortic dissection. J Vasc Surg 2015;61(5): 1192–8.

62. Nienaber CA, Kische S, Rousseau H, et al. Endovascular repair of type B aortic dissection: long-term results of the randomized investigation of stent grafts in aortic dissection trial. Circ Cardiovasc Interv 2013;6(4):407–16.

63. Rodriguez JA, Olsen DM, Lucas L, et al. Aortic remodeling after endografting of thoracoabdominal aortic dissection. J Vasc Surg 2008;47(6):1188–94.

64. Huptas S, Mehta RH, Kühl H, et al. Aortic remodeling in type B aortic dissection: effects of endovascular stent-graft repair and medical treatment on true and false lumen volumes. J Endovasc Ther 2009;16(1):28–38.

65. Lombardi JV, Cambria RP, Nienaber CA, et al. Aortic remodeling after endovascular treatment of complicated type B aortic dissection with the use of a composite device design. J Vasc Surg 2014; 59(6):1544–54.

66. Brunkwall J, Kasprzak P, Verhoeven E, et al. Endovascular repair of acute uncomplicated aortic type B dissection promotes aortic remodelling: 1 year results of the ADSORB trial. Eur J Vasc Endovasc Surg 2014;48(3):285–91.

67. Sigman MM, Palmer OP, Ham SW, et al. Aortic morphologic findings after thoracic endovascular aortic repair for type B aortic dissection. JAMA Surg 2014;149(9):977–83.

68. Luebke T, Brunkwall J. Type B aortic dissection: a review of prognostic factors and meta-analysis of treatment options. Aorta (Stamford) 2014;2(6): 265–78.

69. Kato M, Bai H, Sato K, et al. Determining surgical indications for acute type B dissection based on enlargement of aortic diameter during the chronic phase. Circulation 1995;92(9 Suppl):II107–12.

70. Marui A, Mochizuki T, Mitsui N, et al. Toward the best treatment for uncomplicated patients with type B acute aortic dissection: a consideration for sound surgical indication. Circulation 1999;100(19 Suppl):II275–80.

71. Onitsuka S, Akashi H, Tayama K, et al. Long-term outcome and prognostic predictors of medically treated acute type B aortic dissections. The Ann Thorac Surg 2004;78(4):1268–73.

72. Kunishige H, Myojin K, Ishibashi Y, et al. Predictors of surgical indications for acute type B aortic dissection based on enlargement of aortic diameter during the chronic phase. Jpn J Thorac Cardiovasc Surg 2006;54(11):477–82.

73. Winnerkvist A, Lockowandt U, Rasmussen E, et al. A prospective study of medically treated acute type B aortic dissection. Eur J Vasc Endovasc Surg 2006;32(4):349–55.

74. Marui A, Mochizuki T, Koyama T, et al. Degree of fusiform dilatation of the proximal descending aorta in type B acute aortic dissection can predict late aortic events. J Thorac Cardiovasc Surg 2007; 134(5):1163–70.

75. Trimarchi S, Jonker FHW, Hutchison S, et al. Descending aortic diameter of 5.5 cm or greater is not an accurate predictor of acute type B aortic dissection. J Thorac Cardiovasc Surg 2011; 142(3):e101–7.

76. Akutsu K, Nejima J, Kiuchi K, et al. Effects of the patent false lumen on the long-term outcome of type B acute aortic dissection. Eur J Cardiothorac Surg 2004;26(2):359–66.

77. Sueyoshi E, Sakamoto I, Hayashi K, et al. Growth rate of aortic diameter in patients with type B aortic dissection during the chronic phase. Circulation 2004;110(11 Suppl 1):II256–61.

78. Sueyoshi E, Sakamoto I, Uetani M. Growth rate of affected aorta in patients with type B partially closed aortic dissection. The Ann Thorac Surg 2009;88(4):1251–7.

79. Tsai TT, Evangelista A, Nienaber CA, et al. Partial thrombosis of the false lumen in patients with acute type B aortic dissection. N Engl J Med 2007; 357(4):349–59.

80. Girish A, Padala M, Kalra K, et al. The impact of intimal tear location and partial false lumen thrombosis in acute type B aortic dissection. The Ann Thorac Surg 2016;102(6):1925–32.

81. Song J-M, Kim S-D, Kim J-H, et al. Long-term predictors of descending aorta aneurysmal change in patients with aortic dissection. J Am Coll Cardiol 2007;50(8):799–804.

82. Tolenaar JL, van Keulen JW, Trimarchi S, et al. Number of entry tears is associated with aortic growth in type B dissections. The Ann Thorac Surg 2013;96(1):39–42.

83. Evangelista A, Salas A, Ribera A, et al. Long-term outcome of aortic dissection with patent false lumen: predictive role of entry tear size and location. Circulation 2012;125(25):3133–41.

84. Tolenaar JL, van Keulen JW, Jonker FHW, et al. Morphologic predictors of aortic dilatation in type B aortic dissection. J Vasc Surg 2013;58(5): 1220–5.

85. Trimarchi S, Eagle KA, Nienaber CA, et al. Importance of refractory pain and hypertension in acute type B aortic dissection: insights from the International Registry of Acute Aortic Dissection (IRAD). Circulation 2010;122(13):1283–9.

86. VIRTUE Registry Investigators. Mid-term outcomes and aortic remodelling after thoracic endovascular repair for acute, subacute, and chronic aortic dissection: the VIRTUE Registry. Eur J Vasc Endovasc Surg 2014;48(4):363–71.

87. Chiesa R, Melissano G, Marrocco-Trischitta MM, et al. Spinal cord ischemia after elective stent-graft repair of the thoracic aorta. J Vasc Surg 2005;42(1):11–7.

88. Arnaoutakis DJ, Arnaoutakis GJ, Beaulieu RJ, et al. Results of adjunctive spinal drainage and/or left subclavian artery bypass in thoracic endovascular aortic repair. Ann Vasc Surg 2014;28(1):65–73.

89. Koschyk DH, Meinertz T, Hofmann T, et al. Value of intravascular ultrasound for endovascular stent-graft placement in aortic dissection and aneurysm. J Card Surg 2003;18(5):471–7.

90. Koschyk DH, Nienaber CA, Knap M, et al. How to guide stent-graft implantation in type B aortic dissection? Comparison of angiography, transesophageal echocardiography, and intravascular ultrasound. Circulation 2005;112(9 Suppl):I260–4.

91. Bartel T, Eggebrecht H, Müller S, et al. Comparison of diagnostic and therapeutic value of transesophageal echocardiography, intravascular ultrasonic imaging, and intraluminal phased-array imaging in aortic dissection with tear in the descending thoracic aorta (type B). Am J Cardiol 2007;99(2):270–4.

92. Rocchi G, Lofiego C, Biagini E, et al. Transesophageal echocardiography-guided algorithm for stent-graft implantation in aortic dissection. J Vasc Surg 2004;40(5):880–5.

93. Schütz W, Gauss A, Meierhenrich R, et al. Transesophageal echocardiographic guidance of thoracic aortic stent-graft implantation. J Endovasc Ther 2002;9(Suppl 2):II14–9.

94. Dong ZH, Fu WG, Wang YQ, et al. Retrograde type A aortic dissection after endovascular stent graft placement for treatment of type B dissection. Circulation 2009;119(5):735–41.

95. Canaud L, Ozdemir BA, Patterson BO, et al. Retrograde aortic dissection after thoracic endovascular aortic repair. Ann Surg 2014;260(2):389–95.

96. Gottardi R, Funovics M, Eggers N, et al. Supra-aortic transposition for combined vascular and endovascular repair of aortic arch pathology. The Ann Thorac Surg 2008;86(5):1524–9.

97. Czerny M, Funovics M, Sodeck G, et al. Long-term results of thoracic endovascular aortic repair in atherosclerotic aneurysms involving the descending aorta. J Thorac Cardiovasc Surg 2010;140(6 Suppl):S179–84 [discussion: S185–90].

98. Schoder M, Grabenwöger M, Hölzenbein T, et al. Endovascular repair of the thoracic aorta necessitating anchoring of the stent graft across the arch vessels. J Thorac Cardiovasc Surg 2006;131(2):380–7.

99. Neuhauser B, Czermak BV, Fish J, et al. Type A dissection following endovascular thoracic aortic stent-graft repair. J Endovasc Ther 2005;12(1):74–81.

100. Neuhauser B, Greiner A, Jaschke W, et al. Serious complications following endovascular thoracic aortic stent-graft repair for type B dissection. Eur J Cardiothorac Surg 2008;33(1):58–63.

101. Kpodonu J, Preventza O, Ramaiah VG, et al. Retrograde type A dissection after endovascular stenting of the descending thoracic aorta. Is the risk real? Eur J Cardiothorac Surg 2008;33(6):1014–8.

102. Lopera JE. The amplatzer vascular plug: review of evolution and current applications. Semin Intervent Radiol 2015;32(04):356–69.

103. Yong XZE, Nixon I, Brooks M. Aortic intimal defect occlusion with dual AMPLATZER plugs. J Vasc Interv Radiol 2016;27(6):866.

104. Kölbel T, Lohrenz C, Kieback A, et al. Distal false lumen occlusion in aortic dissection with a home-made extra-large vascular plug: the candy-plug technique. J Endovasc Ther 2013;20(4):484–9.

105. Ogawa Y, Nishimaki H, Chiba K, et al. Candy-plug technique using an excluder aortic extender for distal occlusion of a large false lumen aneurysm in chronic aortic dissection. J Endovasc Ther 2016;23(3):483–6.

106. Kölbel T, Carpenter SW, Lohrenz C, et al. Addressing persistent false lumen flow in chronic aortic dissection: the knickerbocker technique. J Endovasc Ther 2014;21(1):117–22.

107. Kim T-H, Song S-W, Lee K-H, et al. Effects of false lumen procedures on aorta remodeling of chronic DeBakey IIIb aneurysm. The Ann Thorac Surg 2016;102(6):1941–7.

108. Lansman SL, Hagl C, Fink D, et al. Acute type B aortic dissection: surgical therapy. The Ann Thorac Surg 2002;74(5):S1833–5 [discussion: S1857–63].

109. Trimarchi S, Nienaber CA, Rampoldi V, et al. Role and results of surgery in acute type B aortic dissection: insights from the International Registry of Acute Aortic Dissection (IRAD). Circulation 2006;114(1 Suppl):I357–64.

110. Bozinovski J, Coselli JS. Outcomes and survival in surgical treatment of descending thoracic aorta with acute dissection. The Ann Thorac Surg 2008;85(3):965–70 [discussion: 970–1].

111. Peng W, Peng Z, Chai X, et al. Potential biomarkers for early diagnosis of acute aortic dissection. Heart Lung 2015;44(3):205–8.

112. Rudenick PA, Bijnens BH, Garcia-Dorado D, et al. An in vitro phantom study on the influence of tear size and configuration on the hemodynamics of the lumina in chronic type B aortic dissections. J Vasc Surg 2013;57(2):464–74.e5.

113. François CJ, Markl M, Schiebler ML, et al. Four-dimensional, flow-sensitive magnetic resonance imaging of blood flow patterns in thoracic aortic dissections. J Thorac Cardiovasc Surg 2013; 145(5):1359–66.

114. Lu Q, Feng J, Zhou J, et al. Endovascular repair by customized branched stent-graft: a promising treatment for chronic aortic dissection involving the arch branches. J Thorac Cardiovasc Surg 2015;150(6):1631–8.e5.

115. Scali ST, Feezor RJ, Chang CK, et al. Efficacy of thoracic endovascular stent repair for chronic type B aortic dissection with aneurysmal degeneration. J Vasc Surg 2013;58(1):10–7.e11.

116. Han SM, Kuo EC, Woo K, et al. Remodeling of abdominal aortic branch perfusion after thoracic endovascular aortic repair for aortic dissections. J Vasc Surg 2016;64(4):902–11.

Treatment of Complex Thoracoabdominal Aortic Disease

Eric C. Kuo, MD, Sukgu M. Han, MD*

KEYWORDS

- Thoracoabdominal aortic aneurysm • Thoracoabdominal aortic dissections
- Total visceral debranching • Branched endograft • Fenestrated endograft • Sandwich endograft
- TEVAR • EVAR

KEY POINTS

- Thoracoabdominal aortic aneurysms are increasing in incidence. Rupture is associated with a high rate of morbidity and mortality.
- The historic gold standard of open repair can be performed with low rates of complications at centers of excellence. However, these results are not universally achievable.
- With the advent of endovascular therapy, techniques to mitigate the physiologic stress of open surgery have been developed.
- Hybrid open/endovascular operations are being undertaken with total visceral debranching followed by endografting.
- Totally endovascular procedures are now being performed using fenestrated, branched, and parallel endografts.

INTRODUCTION

Despite significant advances in its diagnosis and treatment in the last 60 years, aortic aneurysms remain a significant source of morbidity and mortality. In the United States, aortic aneurysms were the 17th leading cause of death from 1999 to 2007.[1] In particular, extensive aneurysms affecting both the thoracic and abdominal segments carry poor prognosis when left untreated, with survival as low as 24% of patients surviving 2 years after diagnosis, with one-half of the mortalities owing to rupture.[2,3] The 5-year survival ranges from 13% to 46%.[3] Despite significant advances in both open and endovascular surgical techniques, thoracoabdominal aortic aneurysms (TAAA) continue to be among the most challenging pathologies to both patients and surgeons. In this article, we discuss the various treatment options for complex thoracoabdominal aortic aneurysmal disease, with a particular focus on emerging endovascular technologies and innovative techniques.

Etiology

Aortic aneurysms are defined as a dilatation 1.5 times greater than its normal value. The pathophysiology of aortic aneurysms has been attributed to a variety of etiologies, with the most common being degenerative aneurysms accounting for 82% of aneurysms (**Table 1**). The second most common etiology of TAAA, aneurysmal degeneration of chronic aortic dissections, makes

Disclosure Statement: None.
Division of Vascular Surgery and Endovascular Therapy, Department of Surgery, Keck School of Medicine, University of Southern California, 1520 San Pablo Street, Suite 4300, Los Angeles, CA 90033, USA
* Corresponding author. 1520 San Pablo Street, Suite 4300, Los Angeles, CA 90033.
E-mail address: Sukgu.han@med.usc.edu

Table 1
Incidence of etiologies of TAAA

Etiology	Average Incidence, % (Range)
Degenerative	82 (70–93)
Dissection	17 (4–30)
Marfan syndrome	5 (1.6–10.9)
Ehlers-Danlos syndrome	4
Mycotic	2 (1.1–4.2)
Takayasu arteritis	1.2 (0.9–2.1)
Trauma	0.2 (0.1–1.8)

Adapted from Panneton JM, Hollier LH. Nondissecting thoracoabdominal aortic aneurysms: part I. Ann Vasc Surg 1995;9(5):504; with permission.

up 17% of TAAA.[3] The underlying etiology seems to impact the natural history of TAAA. Compared with degenerative aneurysms, aneurysmal degeneration of chronic dissections carries lower long-term survival and tends to rupture at a smaller diameter.[2,4] Additionally, connective tissue disorders, such as Marfan syndrome, Ehlers-Danlos syndrome, and Loeys-Dietz syndrome, have all been implicated in the early development of aneurysmal disease.[5]

TAAAs vary widely in extent, but can be defined as aneurysmal pathology involving both the thoracic and abdominal aorta. The most widely accepted classification system was developed by Crawford and DeNatale[2] (**Fig. 1**). Extent I TAAAs begin distal to the left subclavian and terminate above the renal arteries. Extent II TAAAs extend below the renal arteries. Extent III TAAAs extend from the midthoracic aorta (about the level of T6) to below the renal arteries. Extent IV TAAAs (complete abdominal aorta) extend from T12 to the iliac bifurcation. Last, extent V TAAAs extend from T6 to the renal arteries.

The extent of the TAAA plays a major role in planning the approach to treatment and in the risk of postoperative complications. For example, an extent IV TAAA can potentially be addressed via a smaller incision, whereas the more extensive TAAAs often require larger or 2 separate incisions entering 2 cavities, greatly increasing complication rates. Specifics regarding treatment modalities are addressed in the remainder of this article.

Presentation and Diagnosis

Because many patients with TAAAs are asymptomatic, diagnosis is often made incidentally on imaging for other presentations, especially with the increase in the use of cross-sectional imaging. In

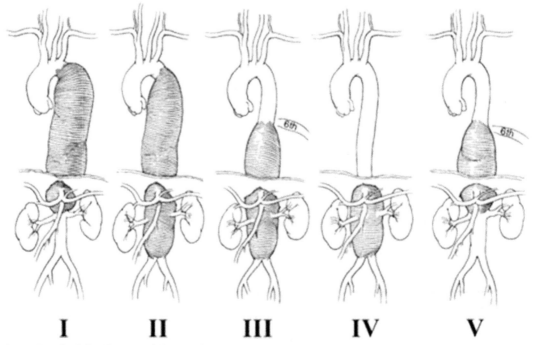

I   II   III   IV   V

Fig. 1. Crawford classification of thoracoabdominal aortic aneurysms. (*From* Huynh TTT, Miller CC III, Estrera AL, et al. Determinants of hospital length of stay after thoracoabdominal aortic aneurysm repair. J Vasc Surg 2002;35(4):649; with permission.)

a review of the TAAA literature, initial presentation was found to be asymptomatic in 43% of patients, symptomatic in 48%, and rupture in 9%.[3] Similar to aneurysms at other arterial segments, the growth rate and rupture risk of TAAA seem to be related to the aneurysm size.[4] When present, symptoms of chest or back pain can signal impending rupture. Mortality rates after rupture range from 40% to 70% for patients who present to hospitals alive, with more than 50% of patients expiring within the first 24 hours postoperatively.[6] The overall mortality rate is likely even higher if those who expire before arrival to the hospital are included.

The high mortality from TAAAs stems from the risk of rupture and subsequent rapid exsanguination. Risk factors for this ill-fated outcome are similar to those in abdominal aortic aneurysms. Chronic obstructive pulmonary disease increases odds of rupture by 3.6.[4] Age is also a strong risk factor, with every decade increase increasing the relative risk by 2.6. Pain, even when nonspecific, was also a significant predictor of rupture, with an odds ratio of 2.3.

Diagnosis is best made with axial imaging; chest radiography has been found to have poor sensitivity and specificity (**Fig. 2**). The gold standard for diagnosis is computed tomography (CT) angiography, ideally electrocardiograph gated, to provide the best imaging of the proximal thoracic aorta. A complete CT scan of the chest, abdomen, and pelvis is essential in evaluating the extent of aneurysmal disease for open operative planning. Additionally, assessment of access vessels is particularly important for endovascular planning.

OPEN REPAIR

Historically, open surgery was the only repair option for TAAAs and is still considered the gold standard for repair and durability.[7] The Crawford classification has proven a useful system for assessing the extent of surgical repair and the associated operative risks. In a large report on 2286 patients undergoing open TAAA repair, the authors reported the highest rates of death (6%), spinal cord deficit (6.3%), and renal failure (8.3%) in extent II (entire thoracoabdominal aortic repair).[8]

Preoperative evaluation of patients under consideration for open TAAA repair is paramount

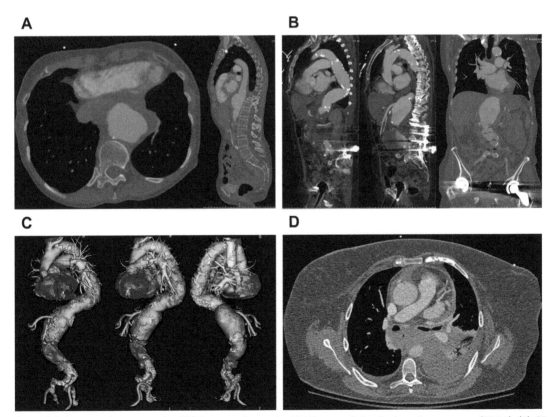

Fig. 2. (*A*) Computed tomography (CT) images of an extent V thoracoabdominal aortic aneurysm (TAAA). (*B*) CT scans of an extent III TAAA. (*C*) Three-dimensional reconstructions of the extent III TAAA shown in (*B*). (*D*) Ruptured TAAA with left hemothorax.

for a good result. Guidelines for evaluation have been published (**Box 1**).

Indications for Repair

The decision to intervene in asymptomatic TAAAs is made based on the risk of rupture against the risk of morbidity and mortality of repair. As the size increases, the risk of rupture rises exponentially.[9] Contrary to infrarenal abdominal aortic aneurysms, there are no level I data supporting a size threshold for repair of TAAAs. A 2010 joint guideline on thoracic aortic disease by multiple societies suggest open repair for TAAA at a threshold of 5.5 cm for patients without significant comorbidities with TAAAs secondary to chronic dissection and endovascular repair for those with degenerative or saccular aneurysms (**Box 2**).

Technique

The location of the aortic pathology dictates the incision location. For extent I and II lesions with disease near the aortic arch, a left fifth interspace incision is usually required (**Fig. 3**). As the aneurysm progresses distally, the incision can be moved accordingly. Ideally, the lowest incision possible should be used, because this placement decreases the risk of pulmonary complications.[10]

Detailed planning regarding aortic branch vessels is required. Based on the extent of disease, visceral, renal, and intercostal arteries may have to be sewn to the graft, with attendant risk of complications to those vascular beds. Involvement down to the iliac arteries presents an additional challenge, because the right iliac artery exposure can be challenging with the standard left-sided incisions. Exposure may require additional mobilization of the distal aorta via division of the inferior mesenteric artery. Last, the course of the ureters over the iliac bifurcation poses an additional risk of injury to these critical structures. Identification can be aided by the preoperative placement of ureteral stents.[10]

Over the past one-half century, the technique of open thoracoabdominal aneurysm repair has been refined. At its core, the procedure consists of replacing the aneurysmal portion of aorta with synthetic or homograft. The proximal anastomosis is completed first, followed by visceral and renal reattachment, usually performed via a Carrel patch directly to the aortic graft (**Fig. 4**). The specific configuration is determined by vessel distances. A large Carrel patch to accommodate widely spaced branches is prone to aneurysmal degeneration.[11] In this situation, multiple branches may be sewn individually to the graft (**Fig. 5**). If occlusive

---

Box 1
Recommendations for preoperative evaluation of patients undergoing thoracic aortic aneurysm repair

Class I

1. In preparation for surgery, imaging studies adequate to establish the extent of disease and the potential limits of the planned procedure are recommended. (Level of evidence: C)

2. Patients with thoracic aortic disease requiring a surgical or catheter-based intervention who have symptoms or other findings of myocardial ischemia should undergo additional studies to determine the presence of significant coronary artery disease. (Level of evidence: C)

3. Patients with unstable coronary syndromes and significant coronary artery disease should undergo revascularization before or at the time of thoracic aortic surgery or endovascular intervention with percutaneous coronary intervention or concomitant coronary artery bypass surgery. (Level of evidence: C)

Class IIa

1. Additional testing is reasonable to quantitate the patient's comorbid states and develop a risk profile. These may include pulmonary function tests, cardiac catheterization, aortography, 24-hour Holter monitoring, noninvasive carotid screening, brain imaging, echocardiography, and neurocognitive testing. (Level of evidence: C)

Class IIb

1. For patients who are to undergo surgery or endovascular intervention for descending thoracic aortic disease, and who have clinically stable, but significant (flow limiting), coronary artery disease, the benefits of coronary revascularization are not well established. (Level of evidence: B)

Data from Hiratzka LF, Bakris GL, Beckman JA, et al. 2010 ACCF/AHA/AATS/ACR/ASA/SCA/SCAI/SIR/STS/SVM guidelines for the diagnosis and management of patients with thoracic aortic disease: executive summary. J Am Coll Cardiol 2010;55(14):1509–44.

> **Box 2**
> **Recommendations for repair of thoracic and thoracoabdominal aortic aneurysms**
>
> *Class I*
>
> 1. For patients with chronic dissection, particularly if associated with a connective tissue disorder, but without significant comorbid disease, and a descending thoracic aortic diameter exceeding 5.5 cm, open repair is recommended. (Level of evidence: B)
>
> 2. For patients with degenerative or traumatic aneurysms of the descending thoracic aorta exceeding 5.5 cm, saccular aneurysms, or postoperative pseudoaneurysms, endovascular stent grafting should be strongly considered when feasible. (Level of evidence: B)
>
> 3. For patients with thoracoabdominal aneurysms, in whom endovascular stent graft options are limited and surgical morbidity is elevated, elective surgery is recommended if the aortic diameter exceeds 6.0 cm, or less if a connective tissue disorder such as Marfan or Loeys-Dietz syndrome is present. (Level of evidence: C)
>
> 4. For patients with thoracoabdominal aneurysms and with end-organ ischemia or significant stenosis from atherosclerotic visceral artery disease, an additional revascularization procedure is recommended. (Level of evidence: B)
>
> *Data from* Hiratzka LF, Bakris GL, Beckman JA, et al. 2010 ACCF/AHA/AATS/ACR/ASA/SCA/SCAI/SIR/STS/SVM guidelines for the diagnosis and management of patients with thoracic aortic disease: executive summary. J Am Coll Cardiol 2010;55(14):1509–44.

disease affects the branches, endarterectomy or bypass may be required before anastomosis. The clamp is then moved distal to the visceral and renal vessels, allowing reperfusion. This maneuver is followed by the distal anastomosis, usually to the iliac arteries.

Coselli and colleagues[12] reported their strategies for open repair after reviewing their outcomes after 1773 consecutive TAAA repairs. Key adjunctive maneuvers in their procedure for all extents include permissive hypothermia (32°C–34°C), moderate systemic heparinization (1 mg/kg), cold perfusion of renal arteries with 4°C crystalloid

solution, and aggressive reattachment of segmental arteries (especially between T8 and L1 for the artery of Adamkiewicz), as well as using sequential aortic clamping when possible. For extent I and II repairs, the authors used cerebral spinal fluid drainage, left heart bypass during the proximal anastomosis, and selective perfusion of the visceral vessels during intercostal and other branch vessel anastomoses.

Extracorporeal circulatory assist
The Crawford technique of TAAA repair involves a simple "clamp and sew" approach. In the hands of

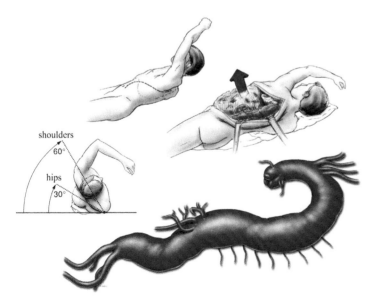

Fig. 3. Patient positioning and incision for an extent II thoracoabdominal aortic aneurysm repair. (*From* Coselli JS, de la Cruz KI, Preventza O, et al. Extent II thoracoabdominal aortic aneurysm repair: how I do it. Semin Thorac Cardiovasc Surg 2016;28(2):225; with permission.)

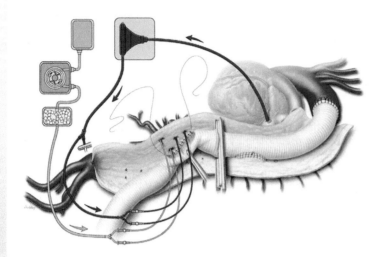

Fig. 4. Extracorporeal circulatory assist, reimplantation of an intercostal artery patch, and anastomosis of renal and visceral Carrel patch. (*From* Coselli JS, de la Cruz KI, Preventza O, et al. Extent II thoracoabdominal aortic aneurysm repair: how I do it. Semin Thorac Cardiovasc Surg 2016;28(2):230; with permission.)

experienced, high-volume surgeons, this technique has been shown to have good results.[13] However, the physiologic stress of cross-clamping the thoracic aorta with subsequent

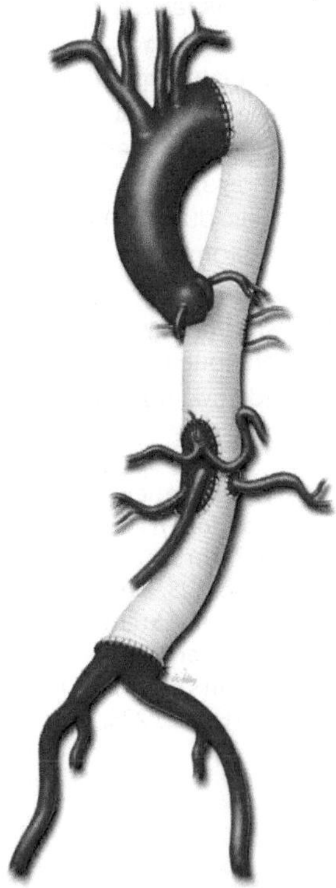

Fig. 5. Surgical repair of an extent II thoracoabdominal aortic aneurysm. The celiac, superior mesenteric, and right renal arteries were reimplanted as a Carrel patch, and the left renal artery was reimplanted separately. (*From* Coselli JS, de la Cruz KI, Preventza O, et al. Extent II thoracoabdominal aortic aneurysm repair: how I do it. Semin Thorac Cardiovasc Surg 2016;28(2):234; with permission.)

ischemia downstream has been mitigated by extracorporeal perfusion. This can be performed in multiple ways, with a common technique being atrial–femoral, with the viscerals and renals being perfused retrograde via a femoral arterial cannula with oxygenated blood taken from the left atrium or pulmonary vein.[14]

For more extensive operations, hypothermic circulatory arrest can be performed on full cardiopulmonary bypass with cooling down to 16°C to 18°C. This procedure serves to protect the end organs during ischemia, but is complicated by coagulopathy and the increased complexity of hypothermic cardiac arrest.

Adjunctive spinal protection

One of the most devastating complications of thoracoabdominal aneurysm repair is spinal cord ischemia, manifested as paraparesis or paraplegia. In a series of 1509 cases, Svensson and colleagues[15] reported an incidence of 16%. As surgical technique has improved with efforts to maintain spinal perfusion with exclusion of the aneurysm, postoperative paraplegia and paraparesis has been reported as low as 5.3% in a recently published series of 3309 TAAA cases.[16] In this large series, reattaching 1 or more pairs of intercostals and lumbar arteries to the graft was done whenever possible.

The spinal cord has multiple collateral arteries feeding it along its course. Proximally, it is supplied by the vertebral arteries, as well as other small branches off the brachiocephalic vessels, such as the internal mammary artery via the intercostals.[17] Moving distally, multiple segmental vessels (intercostal and lumbar arteries) arise directly from the aorta to perfuse the cord. The artery of Adamkiewicz is an important source of perfusion to the cord, often found from T9 to L2 in 75% of cases, and T5 to T8 in 15% of cases.[18] Distally, the spine is supplied by branches of the hypogastric arteries.

Understanding the arterial supply of the spinal cord allows better insight into those patients at greater risk for postoperative neurologic complications. For example, extensive thoracoabdominal aneurysms affecting a large number of intercostals and lumbar arteries, prolonged aortic cross-clamp time, occluded hypogastric arteries, and perioperative hypotension increase the risk of ischemia. These considerations are relevant to all major repairs of the aorta, open or endovascular.

In a review of contemporary spinal cord perfusion strategies, multiple approaches are laid out.[19] Because spinal perfusion pressure is calculated as mean arterial pressure minus cerebral spinal fluid pressure, measures to maximize spinal perfusion include placing a cerebral spinal fluid drain and maintaining a mean arterial pressure of 80 to 100 mm Hg. Similarly, perioperative hypotension has been associated with delayed onset spinal cord ischemia.

The segmental arteries can also be reattached to the graft to improve perfusion. The authors note that vigorously backbleeding arteries are a sign of good collateral flow at that level; those arteries with minimal backbleeding are more important in ischemia prevention. Additionally, these arteries should be clipped or oversewn quickly when identified to prevent loss of perfusion pressure to the network supplying the spinal cord in a "steal" type of phenomenon.

Efforts into identifying spinal cord ischemia before infarction have been made using somatosensory evoked potential and motor evoked potentials. These can be used not only to recognize the onset of ischemia, but can also be used to tailor interventions, that is, finding those segmental arteries most important for perfusion or identifying the minimum required mean arterial pressure. Although conceptually promising, these monitoring techniques can have significant false-positive rates owing to the systemic effects of TAAA as well as surgical and anesthetic maneuvers during repair. Lower body ischemia during aortic cross-clamping will affect the ability of peripheral nerves to transmit signals. These signals can also be affected by intraoperative strokes. Neuromuscular blocking agents can blunt the signals, as can general anesthesia. Furthermore, ischemia localized to the anterior or posterior spinal cord may be missed owing to the orientation of the motor and sensory tracts. Currently, routine neuroelectric monitoring has not been adopted widely.[19]

Outcomes

Experience over the last one-half century in TAAA repairs has resulted in improved outcomes. In a 2007 study of 2286 open TAAA repairs, Coselli and colleagues[8] reported a 30-day survival rate of 95%. Of their patients, 32% experienced pulmonary complications, 7.9% had cardiac events, 5.6% of patients required hemodialysis, 3.8% experienced paraplegia or paraparesis, and 1.7% suffered a stroke. Their results are excellent, especially in light of the fact that 64.2% of their patients underwent extensive repairs for Crawford extent I and II TAAA.

Coselli and colleagues[16] continued their series to 3309 open TAAA repairs. The results were further broken down by Crawford extent as well as age and presentation. Of note, operative mortality was significantly higher in extents II and III (9.5% and 8.8%, respectively) than in extents I and IV (5.9% and 5.4%, respectively). Permanent paraplegia and paraparesis were experienced by 5.3% of patients (although this only affected 1.1% of patients ≤50 years old). Complications were also found to be highest in those patients with extent II repairs.

These outcomes achieved through extensive experience of repairing thousands of patients establish the benchmark results of high-volume centers of excellence. However, more sobering is the statewide study of outcomes after open TAAA repairs in California from 1991 to 2002.[20] In 1010 patients, the observed 30-day overall mortality was 19.2% for elective cases and 48.4% for ruptured cases, with a steep increase in the mortality for every decade in age. This large study is more likely a reflection of real-world experience and results of open TAAA repair, suggesting that these complex operations be preferentially performed at high-volume centers of excellence.

HYBRID REPAIR

The endovascular revolution was pioneered by Parodi and associates in 1991,[21] transforming the field of vascular surgery. Soon after, the technology was quickly adapted for the thoracic aorta with good results.[22] With growing collective experience with endografts, the challenge of complex thoracoabdominal aortic disease was addressed, with the goal to avoid the significant physiologic insult associated with open TAAA repair. This has been approached via hybrid open/endovascular repair, in which the paravisceral aorta is debranched by bypass, creating a segment of aorta that can be relined with a endograft. This allows for lengthening of the landing zone into the paravisceral aorta. The first case of a combined approach was described in 1999.[23] Thereafter, the technique was adopted in many centers worldwide, especially owing to the perceived benefits of such a procedure being lower morbidity owing to the avoidance of a thoracotomy, aortic cross-clamping, single lung ventilation, and extended organ ischemia.[24]

Indications

Indications for hybrid operation include patients who would be poor candidates for extensive open TAAA repair, especially patients with advanced age or severe comorbidities. Although some have preferentially used hybrid technique over open repair owing to the perceived benefit in the safety profile, hybrid procedures are still major operations. Patients should be evaluated thoroughly and have their preexisting medical conditions optimized. Patients with chronic obstructive pulmonary disease may be particularly well-suited for a hybrid procedure because this technique avoids the pulmonary morbidity of a thoracotomy with diaphragm incision. A detailed abdominal surgical history is required, because that may affect choice of approach to avoid extensive intraperitoneal or retroperitoneal adhesions.

Preoperative planning should include a careful radiologic examination of the thoracic aorta and the visceral and renal branches, as well as the iliacs. Because patients are undergoing treatment for TAAA, the inflow for the bypass is most often retrograde from the iliacs. Patients with proximal flow-limiting dissections or severe aortoiliac occlusive disease may be poor candidates for debranching.

Technique

The wide array of aortic pathology and anatomy allows for a variety of bypass techniques to be used. Exposure can be performed via a midline transabdominal or retroperitoneal incision. Inflow is commonly the common iliac artery, but in the presence of occlusive disease, the infrarenal aorta or previously placed grafts can also be used.[25] In patients with significant aortoiliac occlusive disease, antegrade flow can be obtained from the hepatic or splenic artery.[26] Prosthetic conduits for bypass are available in an assortment of configurations, from individual bypasses to premade trifurcated grafts with a jump graft. To avoid kinking, retrograde grafts are laid in "lazy C" configuration (**Fig. 6**). To prevent type 2 endoleaks in the subsequent endograft deployment, end-to-end anastomoses can be performed for each branch. Alternatively, anastomoses can be performed in

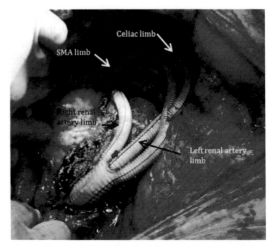

Fig. 6. Total abdominal aortic debranching with trifurcated Dacron grafts to the renal and visceral arteries. Note the "lazy C" configuration to avoid kinking. SMA, superior mesenteric artery.

an end-to-side configuration. In this setting, the native vessel must be ligated proximal to the anastomosis.

After the open debranching procedure, endovascular graft placement may be performed in concomitant or staged fashion. A staged approach allows the patients to recover from the stress of a major visceral and renal reconstruction. However, in patients with large TAAA, the waiting period also leaves the patient at risk for interval rupture. There have been reports of interval mortalities from rupture—3 patients died of rupture while waiting a mean of 20 days after debranching.[27]

Single stage procedures are necessary in emergent situations and are facilitated by direct vascular access to deploy the graft. However, with the long operative times of total abdominal debranching, the additional time needed to deploy the graft and the increased risk for contrast-induced nephropathy need to be taken into consideration. With these constraints in mind, staged procedures may be better for patients with significant comorbidities and extensive TAAA disease and single stage procedures for those patients with prohibitively large risk for rupture (**Fig. 7**).[24]

Outcomes

Outcomes of hybrid procedures have been promising in multiple case series. Fulton and colleagues[26] reported results of 13 visceral bypasses in 10 patients with no perioperative mortality, neurologic deficits, coagulopathy, or renal dysfunction. However, 1 patient suffered a

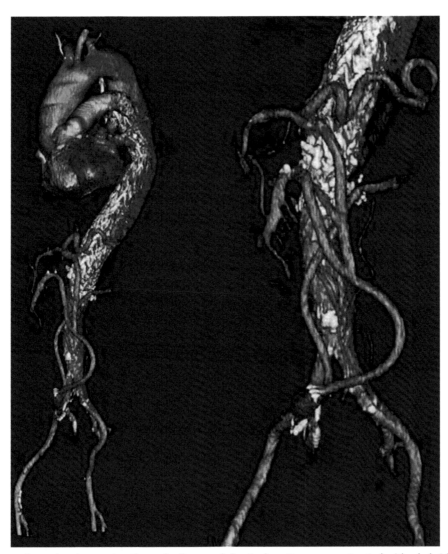

Fig. 7. Three-dimensional reconstructions of a thoracoabdominal aortic aneurysm treated with a hybrid open/endovascular procedure. Note the graft arising from the right common iliac artery supplying the abdominal aortic branches.

myocardial infarction and 2 developed pneumonia. On a mean follow-up of 8.7 months, all bypass grafts were found to be patent.

In a larger series by Ham and colleagues,[25] 124 bypasses were performed in 51 patients. The authors reported a 30-day and in-hospital mortality rate of 3.9% (2 patients)—one expired from bowel ischemia after visceral/renal debranching for a symptomatic extent II TAAA, and the other patient from ruptured arch aneurysm despite debranching and concomitant endovascular repair. Thirty-nine percent of patients experienced major postoperative complications, with 8% experiencing pulmonary and renal complications, temporary paraplegia in 1 patient (no spinal drain was placed

preoperatively owing to urgency), and stroke in 2 patients. Bypass graft patency seems to be excellent, with a primary patency of 95.3% at 1 and 3 years in that series.

These 2 single-center studies demonstrated excellent results, especially regarding mortality and paralysis. A metaanalysis of combined open endovascular techniques of 14 studies was performed in 2012.[24] The authors found a pooled rate for 30-day and in-hospital mortality of 14.3%, symptomatic spinal cord ischemia 7%, with irreversible paraplegia 4.4%, permanent renal failure 7%, and mesenteric ischemia 4.5%. Pooled estimates for primary technical success and visceral graft patency were 95.4% and 96.5%, respectively. The investigators concluded that, despite the less invasive nature of a hybrid procedure, patients who are selected for this operation are often limited by severe comorbidities that place them at high risk for complications. High-volume centers consistently show better results with the treatment of this complex disease process.

TOTAL ENDOVASCULAR REPAIR OF THORACOABDOMINAL AORTIC PATHOLOGY

Despite the intuitive benefits of a hybrid approach, complication rates remain high owing to the comorbidities of the patient population. This finding has been the impetus to develop totally endovascular approaches to the repair of complex thoracoabdominal aortic disease. As endovascular technology has progressed, pioneers in the field have devised a wide variety of solutions to this difficult problem.

The main challenge in total endovascular repair of a thoracoabdominal aorta is maintaining perfusion of the visceral and renal arteries while achieving complete exclusion of the aneurysm. The options for aortic branch incorporation are in the form of intraluminal bridging to branch stents such as fenestrated, branch cuff endografts, or that of parallel grafting where the branch stents run outside the aortic endograft in parallel fashion.

Fenestrated, Branched Endografts

Reinforced fenestrations are essentially small holes tailored to the size of the branch vessel reinforced with radiopaque wire for cannulation assistance and seal. They are typically used when the branches are located within the seal zone, where the aortic endografts appose the aortic wall. These are often reinforced with a stent placed through the fenestration to stabilize the alignment.

Branched endovascular repair takes this concept a step further by joining a small, covered stent to the main body endograft, creating a branch cuff. This configuration increases the amount of seal zone available to the branch artery stent. Depending on the device, these sidearm branches can come precannulated, allowing for easy snaring from brachial access at the time of procedure. Currently, access to these fenestrated, branched endografts for TAAAs in the United States remains limited to centers with investigational device exemption protocols.

The Cook custom-made devices and t-Branch device (Cook Medical, Bloomington, IN) have been used with excellent midterm results.[28] The custom-made devices are specifically tailored for each patient's aortic anatomy and can take 6 to 8 weeks for manufacture. With this significant constraint, the goal has been to create off-the-shelf grafts that have the flexibility to address most patients. The t-Branch is one such device with 4 caudally directed external cuffs (**Fig. 8**). The radial orientation of the branch cuffs has been based on the anatomic study of aortic branch distribution of previously studied patients.

The Gore Excluder thoracoabdominal graft (W. L. Gore Inc, Flagstaff, AZ) is based on its infrarenal graft. It is also an off-the-shelf, 4 branched endograft, with 4 caudally directed branches (**Fig. 9**). The branch portals can be prewired for ease of access. The conformability of the main body endograft seems to be promising.

The Medtronic device (Medtronic Vascular, Santa Rosa, CA) takes a somewhat different approach to this problem, with a bifurcated main body, with 1 leg expanding into a manifold for the 4 visceral vessels and the other leading to the infrarenal aorta, which can then be mated to a standard infra renal bifurcated device (**Fig. 10**).

Indications

Consideration of a full endovascular repair should be given to patients with extensive previous thoracic or abdominal operations, where scar tissue in a redo field may significantly increase the complexity of the procedure. Moreover, patients with significant comorbidities should also be evaluated for endovascular repair.

Ideally, the portion of the aorta with branches to be incorporated into the graft should be relatively straight. This enables the graft to be maneuvered more easily to line up the fenestrations with the branches in that segment. A large aneurysm sac enables easier adjustment for alignment in all dimensions. After alignment, the individual fenestration then target branches will need to be cannulated. As such, significant stenosis can make cannulation extremely challenging and would be considered a contraindication to fenestrated repair.

As the technology matures, the indications for complete endovascular repair will likely expand to include even those patients who would otherwise be good candidates for open repair. The less invasive nature and quicker recovery amount to an attractive proposition for both surgeon and patient.

Technique

As with other complex endovascular procedures, close review of preoperative CT angiography of the chest, abdomen, and pelvis is mandatory. Centerline flow reconstruction is the most accurate way to determine sizing as well as identify

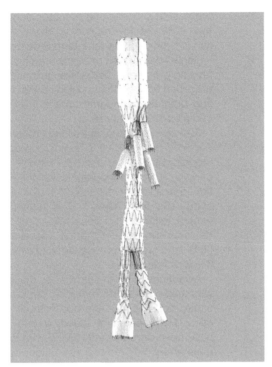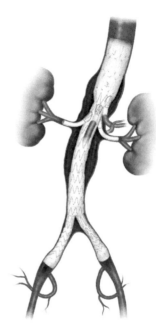

Fig. 8. Cook t-Branch device. (*Courtesy of* Cook Medical, Bloomington, IN; with permission.)

branch locations. Commonly, a "clock" reference is used to denote radial orientation of the aortic branch vessels.

The main body of the graft is introduced through a femoral access. The branch cuffs and fenestrations are accessed through the brachial or contralateral femoral approach, depending on the orientation of the branch vessels.[29] The brachial access is commonly used for catheterization of the celiac and superior mesenteric artery, but can also be very useful for any branch with severe caudal orientation.

After this access is achieved, the main body of the endograft is deployed into the aneurysm, still partially constrained to allow rotation and cranial–caudal movement for alignment. The branches are then cannulated individually. At this point, the main body device is fully deployed. Balloon-expandable or self-expanding stents are then deployed to bridge the main body and the target vessel. Any additional necessary distal or extensions of the endograft are then placed, depending on the extent of disease. Alternatively, the implantation sequence can be modified to restore pelvic circulation earlier. In this technique, the branched main body is fully deployed, distal extensions completed, and the large delivery sheath is completely withdrawn to reperfuse the

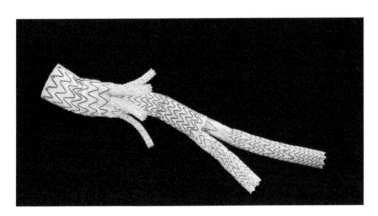

Fig. 9. Gore excluder thoracoabdominal graft. (*Courtesy of* W.L. Gore & Associates, Inc, Newark, DE; with permission.)

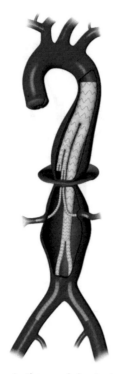

Fig. 10. Medtronic thoracoabdominal device. (*Courtesy of* Medtronic, Jacksonville, FL; with permission.)

internal iliac artery. This maneuver is followed by individual branch stenting from the brachial approach. Reestablishing flow to the internal iliac arteries preserves an important collateral circulation to the spinal cord.[30]

Branched endografts have several advantages over simple fenestrated devices. In addition to providing a greater seal zone, the cranial–caudal orientation of the cuffs enable a smoother transition between the main body and the endografts. This potentially decreases the risk of endoleaks, stent fracture, and kinking. However, the use of branched endografts is limited to those aneurysms with a large diameter near the branches, because compression between the main body and the aortic wall may cause occlusion. Another benefit to branched endografts is the possibility of a staged procedure, not to be taken lightly given the extensive fluoroscopy time and contrast administration during these complex cases. The main body can be deployed with the branches providing flow into the branches. This advantage must be balanced with continued sac pressurization during the interim period, arguably a higher risk for rupture owing to loss of outflow.[29]

Outcomes

The midterm results of these interventions have been promising, with multiple studies reporting procedural success and branch patency of more than 90% with low rates of morbidity and mortality.[31–37] Although no long-term data are available, multiple reviews and metaanalyses have reported favorable midterm outcomes of fenestrated and branched endografts, concluding that fenestrated and branched endografts are a viable option in complex TAAA disease.

A review of 7 studies treating 155 patients with TAAA[36] reported 94.2% technical success, 7.1% mortality at 30 days, and 3.2% paraplegia or paraparesis. These encouraging results were reaffirmed in a recent metaanalysis of multibranched endografts for TAAAs.[37] The authors found a pooled technical success rate of 98.9%, a 30-day mortality of 9%, target vessel patency of 98%, and spinal cord ischemia of 17%, of which 6% was irreversible.

Avoidance of open surgery has the intuitive advantages of reduced morbidity, but these complicated approaches are not without their own risks. Retroperitoneal bleeding and mortalities have been reported after guide wire injury to the renal artery.[32,33] Another risk unique to endovascular treatment is iatrogenic dissection—mortality owing to dissection of all 4 visceral arteries has been reported.[37]

Physician-Modified Endovascular Grafts

Although the worldwide experience of manufactured custom, off-the-shelf fenestrated, and branched devices includes hundreds of patients with midterm follow-up, these devices are not currently commercially available in the United States. Even at select centers with investigational device exemption protocols, both custom and standard devices take several weeks to manufacture and deliver.[38] Often, patients with excessively large aneurysms are at a prohibitive risk of rupture during this time frame. Furthermore, patients presenting with rupture also do not stand to benefit from this technology. To address this issue, the creation of physician-modified endografts has been reported.

Indications

Physician-modified endografts allow for the creation of fenestrated and branched endografts by the treating physicians at the time of the implantation. Thus, physician-modified endografts are used in patients whose comorbidities preclude open surgery with an urgent need for repair. The main concern for physician-modified endografts is the lack of manufacturing quality control, as well as an increased risk of contamination once the devices are altered. A number of physicians have reported their experience with physician-modified endografts through investigational device exemption protocol, whereas others perform physician-modified endografts for compassionate use in patients requiring urgent repair who do not have other treatment options.

Technique

The most essential part is precise preoperative planning and modification, using high-resolution CT angiography with centerline reconstruction. Oderich and Ricotta[39] published their technique for physician-modified endografts in 2009. The Cook Zenith is the most common base platform device of choice in the literature. A key feature of the device is that it can be partially deployed, modified, then resheathed for deployment with constraining wires in place for intraaortic positioning. Fenestrations are created with fine-tipped cautery and reinforced with radiopaque wire. Branch cuffs can also be incorporated (**Fig. 11**). At this point, the deployment of the device and cannulation of the branches is similar to a prefabricated endograft, with similar results.

Outcomes

The early and midterm results of physician-modified endografts have been promising. Starnes and Tatum[40] reported a series of 26 patients with 63 fenestrations created, with no major adverse events and 100% technical success. This technique has been used in a series of patients presenting with acute aortic syndromes.[41] These outstanding results should be viewed in light of the fact that the series included para and juxtarenal aneurysms as well as the true TAAA. The authors reported a technical success rate of 92%, a 30-day mortality of 19%, and a spinal cord ischemia rate of 14%. One-year branch patency stood at 98%,[41] establishing this as a viable option for patients in grave situations, especially when taking into account the rates of morbidity and mortality of previous studies on open repairs.[20]

Parallel Endografts

Parallel endografts use commercially available endovascular components to treat TAAAs. First devised as a bail out maneuver to preserve renal

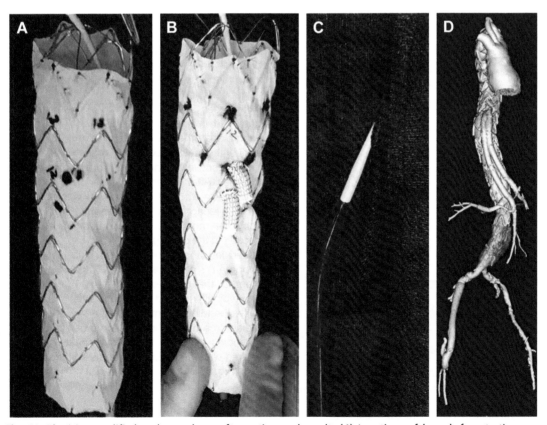

Fig. 11. Physician-modified endovascular graft creation and result. (*A*) Locations of branch fenestrations are marked. (*B*) Fenestrations are created and branch cuffs sewn on. (*C*) The endograft is completely resheathed into original delivery device. (*D*) Computed tomography reconstruction of a thoracoabdominal aortic aneurysm status post repair with a physician-modified endovascular graft.

artery perfusion in inadvertently high deployment of infrarenal endograft,[42] the concept has been refined first in juxtarenal aneurysms and expanded to include treatment of TAAA. Parallel endografts refer to multiple endografts placed in parallel within the same lumen, directing flow in multiple directions. The proximal seal of the main body can thus cover the branch vessel orifice while maintaining perfusion via covered stent running parallel to the main body (**Fig. 12**). They have been referred to as chimneys, periscopes, and snorkels. Chimneys and snorkels have inflow antegrade, and periscopes have retrograde inflow.

The Achilles heel of parallel grafting is the unavoidable creation of a gutter. The potential space between 2 parallel endografts is referred to as a gutter (**Fig. 13**). To minimize gutter leak, adequate overlap and sizing must be obtained, so that any gutter present will thrombose owing to low flow. In an in vitro study, the ideal endograft oversizing in the parallel stent technique was 30%, obtaining minimal gutters, stent compression, and infolding.[43]

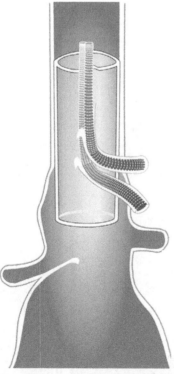

Fig. 12. Parallel grafting. The celiac and superior mesenteric arteries are perfused via "snorkel" endografts running in parallel to the main aortic device. (*From* Tolenaar JL, Zandvoort HJA, Hazenberg CEVB, et al. The double two-chimney technique for complete renovisceral revascularization in a suprarenal aneurysm. J Vasc Surg 2013;58(2):479; with permission.)

To avoid excessively long parallel grafts to provide inflow to visceral vessels in TAAA, a sandwich technique has been described.[44] A proximal seal in the thoracic aorta is achieved with an endograft, which provides a new aortic lumen in which to deploy parallel grafts to provide branch vessel perfusion. Essentially, the chimney grafts are "sandwiched" between 2 aortic endografts (**Fig. 14**).

Indications

Indications for parallel endografting are similar to those of fenestrated and branched endografts, namely, complex aortic pathology in patients not amenable to major open operations. Additionally, this technique has advantages in patients with severely angulated aortic segments and stenosis of target vessels not amenable to commercially available endografts. Contraindications include narrow aortic lumens from stenosis, and certain dissections where the compressed lumen would not allow enough space for all parallel components.

Technique

Special consideration is given to the size of and the distance of the origins of the branch vessels to the proximal extent of the endograft. Access to the bilateral femoral artery and at least 1 brachial artery are usually required. Of utmost importance is maintaining wire purchase into the target vessels.

In cases of TAAA, the proximal endograft deployed in the thoracic aorta,[44] taking care to ensure that the distal extent of the graft lands above the celiac axis. The branch vessels are then selectively cannulated from the upper extremities. After this, the remainder of the aneurysm is treated with another endograft with at least a 5-cm overlap.[44] To minimize gutters, the distal endograft must be larger than the proximal. Before deploying the distal graft, covered stents are introduced into the branch vessels. The distal aortic endograft is then deployed, followed by deployment of the covered stents. The branch stents are typically relined with additional bare metal self-expanding stents to better withstand the radial force of the thoracic aortic devices. TAAAs extending down to the iliac bifurcation can be treated with an additional standard bifurcated device (**Fig. 15**).

Outcomes

Overall, short-term results from parallel grafting have been encouraging. Most of the parallel grafting literature pertains to the treatment of pararenal, juxtarenal aortic aneurysms. For the treatment of pararenal aortic pathologies, a

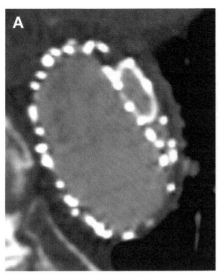 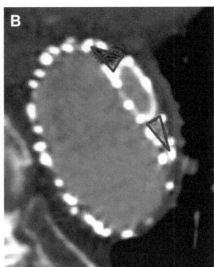

Fig. 13. (A) Computed tomographic image of parallel grafts. (B) The "gutters" are demarcated by the red triangles.

systematic review with 123 patients comparing fenestrated and parallel endografts found no differences in terms of 30-day mortality, renal impairment, or endoleak.[45]

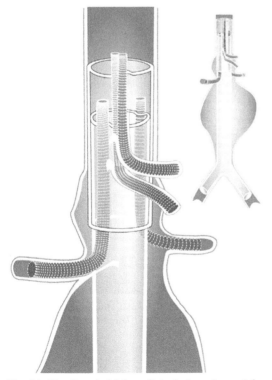

Fig. 14. The "sandwich" graft technique is used for complete repair. The parallel grafts for the renal arteries are placed between 2 aortic endografts. (*From* Tolenaar JL, Zandvoort HJA, Hazenberg CEVB, et al. The double two-chimney technique for complete renovisceral revascularization in a suprarenal aneurysm. J Vasc Surg 2013;58(2):479; with permission.)

Specifically looking at the outcomes of parallel grafts, Wilson and colleagues[46] performed a systemic review of all periscope grafts for endovascular aneurysm repair, with 176 patients with abdominal aneurysms and 58 with thoracoabdominal aneurysms. The investigators reported a 30-day mortality rate of 5.1%, type 1 endoleak rate of 11.5%, and a 1.9% branch vessel occlusion rate at a mean follow-up of 12 months. Although short-term in follow-up, these data support the continued use of this graft configuration in patients with anatomy unsuitable for more conventional devices.

Further evaluation in multicenter studies supported early results.[47,48] The largest of these was the PERICLES study (Programme of Investigation in Cardiovascular Diseases), with 898 chimney grafts placed in 517 patients. Their outcomes were similar in success—with a primary patency rate of 94%. However, their survival at a mean follow-up of 17 months was 79%, which the authors attributed to the high-risk nature of these patients who were not candidates for open operations. Additionally, significant sac regression was found.[47] Similar to fenestrated and branched endografts, the literature on parallel endografts is dominated by pararenal and juxtarenal aneurysms, making the assessment of its efficacy on TAAA difficult.

A key limitation of emerging endovascular technology is the lack of long-term follow-up at this point. An assortment of endovascular techniques is being used to address the gamut of aortic pathology with no established, standardized protocols to allow rigorous evaluation. There are no manufacturer instructions for use for these applications. Often, stents and grafts from multiple

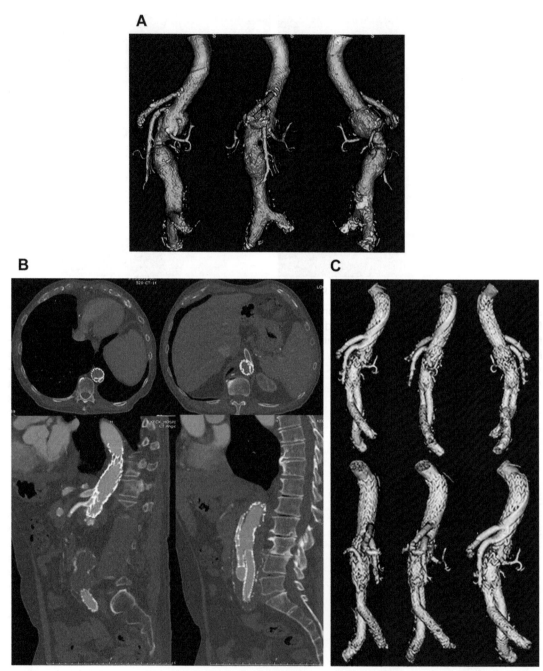

Fig. 15. (*A*) Three-dimensional reconstruction of a paravisceral aortic aneurysm. (*B*) Axial and sagittal computed tomography images of celiac and superior mesenteric artery parallel endografts. (*C*) Three-dimensional reconstruction of totally endovascular repair with parallel endografts.

manufacturers are used together in previously untested applications.

Although the enthusiasm over these new procedures is appropriately high, there have been reports suggesting caution in widespread adoption. The increased number of modules in the repair adds additional points of failure and endoleak.

Chaudhuri and colleagues[49] reported a case of a thoracic aortic aneurysm repaired with chimney graft to the left subclavian artery, which dislocated with continued pressurization and growth of the sac, which required relining. The authors suggest a longer overlap, 5 cm, instead of the 2 cm in the instructions for use for Viabahn stents. Notably, at this point there are no instructions for use regarding the use of these stents in a parallel configuration.

In a single-center experience with parallel grafts, Scali and colleagues[50] reported good success with the technique, but did so with the caveat that there may be a higher rate of endoleak (32%) and lower branch patency rate (88% at 1 year and 85% at 3 years) than previously reported.

Parallel grafts, especially in the "sandwich" technique, offer an additional challenge when it comes to reintervention. It is difficult enough to cannulate a fenestration or graft branch during the initial procedure, cannulating the orifice of a 6-mm Viabahn stent in between 2 thoracic aortic devices raises this technical challenge even further.

SUMMARY

Although open repair remains the gold standard treatment of TAAAs, outstanding results remain achievable only at high-volume centers of excellence. Innovations in endovascular devices as well as technique are expanding treatment indications for TAAAs. As more complex branched, fenestrated devices become available, greater levels of sophistication in imaging analysis and technical skills are required in treating physicians. More work remains to be done to evaluate the mid-term and long-term results of these approaches to complex thoracoabdominal aortic disease, but the future is promising.

REFERENCES

1. National Center for Injury Prevention, Control. WISQARS leading causes of death reports, 1999-2007. CDC Website. Available at: https://webappa.cdc.gov/sasweb/ncipc/leadcaus10.html. Accessed September 11, 2016.
2. Crawford ES, DeNatale RW. Thoracoabdominal aortic aneurysm: observations regarding the natural course of the disease. J Vasc Surg 1986;3(4):578–82.
3. Panneton JM, Hollier LH. Nondissecting thoracoabdominal aortic aneurysms: part I. Ann Vasc Surg 1995;9(5):503–14.
4. Griepp RB, Ergin MA, Galla JD, et al. Natural history of descending thoracic and thoracoabdominal aneurysms. Ann Thorac Surg 1999;67(6):1927–30 [discussion: 1953–8].
5. Hiratzka LF, Bakris GL, Beckman JA, et al. 2010 ACCF/AHA/AATS/ACR/ASA/SCA/SCAI/SIR/STS/SVM guidelines for the diagnosis and management of patients with thoracic aortic disease: executive summary. J Am Coll Cardiol 2010;55(14):1509–44.
6. Cowan JA Jr, Dimick JB, Wainess RM, et al. Ruptured thoracoabdominal aortic aneurysm treatment in the United States: 1988 to 1998. J Vasc Surg 2003;38(2):319–22.
7. Coselli JS. Update on repairs of the thoracoabdominal aorta. Tex Heart Inst J 2013;40(5):572–4.
8. Coselli JS, Bozinovski J, LeMaire SA. Open surgical repair of 2286 thoracoabdominal aortic aneurysms. Ann Thorac Surg 2007;83(2):S862–4 [discussion: S890–2].
9. Davies RR, Goldstein LJ, Coady MA, et al. Yearly rupture or dissection rates for thoracic aortic aneurysms: simple prediction based on size. Ann Thorac Surg 2002;73(1):17–28.
10. Acher CW, Wynn M. Thoracic and thoracoabdominal aneurysms: open surgical treatment. Rutherford's Vasc Surg 2014.
11. Dardik A, Perler BA, Roseborough GS, et al. Aneurysmal expansion of the visceral patch after thoracoabdominal aortic replacement: an argument for limiting patch size? J Vasc Surg 2001;34(3):405–10.
12. Coselli JS, Conklin LD, LeMaire SA. Thoracoabdominal aortic aneurysm repair: review and update of current strategies. Ann Thorac Surg 2002;74(5):S1881–4 [discussion: S1892–8].
13. Patel VI, Ergul E, Conrad MF, et al. Continued favorable results with open surgical repair of type IV thoracoabdominal aortic aneurysms. J Vasc Surg 2011;53(6):1492–8.
14. Conrad MF, Ergul EA, Patel VI, et al. Evolution of operative strategies in open thoracoabdominal aneurysm repair. J Vasc Surg 2011;53(5):1195–201.e1.
15. Svensson LG, Crawford ES, Hess KR, et al. Experience with 1509 patients undergoing thoracoabdominal aortic operations. J Vasc Surg 1993;17(2):357–68 [discussion: 368–70].
16. Coselli JS, LeMaire SA, Preventza O, et al. Outcomes of 3309 thoracoabdominal aortic aneurysm repairs. J Thorac Cardiovasc Surg 2016;151(5):1323–38.
17. Griepp RB, Griepp EB. Spinal cord perfusion and protection during descending thoracic and thoracoabdominal aortic surgery: the collateral network concept. Ann Thorac Surg 2007;83(2):S865–9 [discussion: S890–2].
18. Lazorthes G, Gouaze A, Zadeh JO, et al. Arterial vascularization of the spinal cord. Recent studies of the anastomotic substitution pathways. J Neurosurg 1971;35(3):253–62.
19. Etz CD, Weigang E, Hartert M, et al. Contemporary spinal cord protection during thoracic and thoracoabdominal aortic surgery and endovascular aortic repair: a position paper of the vascular domain of the European Association for Cardio-Thoracic surgery†. Eur J Cardiothorac Surg 2015;47(6):943–57.
20. Rigberg DA, McGory ML, Zingmond DS, et al. Thirty-day mortality statistics underestimate the risk of repair

of thoracoabdominal aortic aneurysms: a statewide experience. J Vasc Surg 2006;43(2):217–22.

21. Parodi JC, Palmaz JC, Barone HD. Transfemoral intraluminal graft implantation for abdominal aortic aneurysms. Ann Vasc Surg 1991;5(6):491–9.

22. Dake MD, Miller DC, Semba CP. Transluminal placement of endovascular stent-grafts for the treatment of descending thoracic aortic aneurysms. N Engl J Med 1994;331(26):1729–34.

23. Quiñones-Baldrich WJ, Panetta TF, Vescera CL, et al. Repair of type IV thoracoabdominal aneurysm with a combined endovascular and surgical approach. J Vasc Surg 1999;30(3):555–60.

24. Moulakakis KG, Mylonas SN, Antonopoulos CN, et al. Combined open and endovascular treatment of thoracoabdominal aortic pathologies: a systematic review and meta-analysis. Ann Cardiothorac Surg 2012;1(3):267–76.

25. Ham SW, Chong T, Moos J, et al. Arch and visceral/renal debranching combined with endovascular repair for thoracic and thoracoabdominal aortic aneurysms. J Vasc Surg 2011;54(1):30–41.

26. Fulton JJ, Farber MA, Marston WA, et al. Endovascular stent-graft repair of pararenal and type IV thoracoabdominal aortic aneurysms with adjunctive visceral reconstruction. J Vasc Surg 2005;41(2):191–8.

27. Drinkwater SL, Böckler D, Eckstein H, et al. The visceral hybrid repair of thoraco-abdominal aortic aneurysms – a collaborative approach. Eur J Vasc Endovasc Surg 2009;38(5):578–85.

28. Reilly LM, Rapp JH, Grenon SM, et al. Efficacy and durability of endovascular thoracoabdominal aortic aneurysm repair using the caudally directed cuff technique. J Vasc Surg 2012;56(1):53–64.

29. Ricotta JJ, Oderich GS. Fenestrated and branched stent grafts. Perspect Vasc Surg Endovasc Ther 2008;20(2):174–87 [discussion: 188–9].

30. Maurel B, Delclaux N, Sobocinski J, et al. Editor's Choice – the impact of early pelvic and lower limb reperfusion and attentive peri-operative management on the incidence of spinal cord ischemia during thoracoabdominal aortic aneurysm endovascular repair. Eur J Vasc Endovasc Surg 2015;49(3):248–54.

31. Haulon S, Amiot S, Magnan PE, et al. An analysis of the French multicentre experience of fenestrated aortic endografts: medium-term outcomes. Ann Surg 2010;251(2):357–62.

32. Chuter TAM, Rapp JH, Hiramoto JS, et al. Endovascular treatment of thoracoabdominal aortic aneurysms. J Vasc Surg 2008;47(1):6–16.

33. Kristmundsson T, Sonesson B, Malina M, et al. Fenestrated endovascular repair for juxtarenal aortic pathology. J Vasc Surg 2009;49(3):568–75.

34. Muhs BE, Verhoeven ELG, Zeebregts CJ, et al. Midterm results of endovascular aneurysm repair with branched and fenestrated endografts. J Vasc Surg 2006;44(1):9–15.

35. Tambyraja AL, Fishwick NG, Bown MJ, et al. Fenestrated aortic endografts for juxtarenal aortic aneurysm: medium term outcomes. Eur J Vasc Endovasc Surg 2011;42(1):54–8.

36. Bakoyiannis CN, Economopoulos KP. Fenestrated and branched endografts for the treatment of thoracoabdominal aortic aneurysms: a systematic review. J Endovasc Ther 2010;17:201–9.

37. Hu Z, Li Y, Peng R, et al. Multibranched stent-grafts for the treatment of thoracoabdominal aortic aneurysms a systematic review and meta-analysis. J Endovasc Ther 2016;23(4):626–33.

38. Fernandez CC, Sobel JD, Gasper WJ, et al. Standard off-the-shelf versus custom-made multibranched thoracoabdominal aortic stent grafts. J Vasc Surg 2016;63(5):1208–15.

39. Oderich GS, Ricotta JJ. Modified fenestrated stent grafts: device design, modifications, implantation, and current applications. Perspect Vasc Surg Endovasc Ther 2009;21(3):157–67.

40. Starnes BW, Tatum B. Early report from an investigator-initiated investigational device exemption clinical trial on physician-modified endovascular grafts. J Vasc Surg 2013;58(2):311–7.

41. Sweet MP, Starnes BW, Tatum B. Endovascular treatment of thoracoabdominal aortic aneurysm using physician-modified endografts. J Vasc Surg 2015; 62(5):1160–7.

42. Greenberg RK, Clair D, Srivastava S, et al. Should patients with challenging anatomy be offered endovascular aneurysm repair? J Vasc Surg 2003;38(5): 990–6.

43. Mestres G, Uribe JP, García-Madrid C, et al. The best conditions for parallel stenting during EVAR: an in vitro study. Eur J Vasc Endovasc Surg 2012; 44(5):468–73.

44. Lobato AC, Camacho-Lobato L. A new technique to enhance endovascular thoracoabdominal aortic aneurysm therapy—the sandwich procedure. Semin Vasc Surg 2012;25(3):153–60.

45. Donas KP, Eisenack M, Panuccio G, et al. The role of open and endovascular treatment with fenestrated and chimney endografts for patients with juxtarenal aortic aneurysms. J Vasc Surg 2012;56(2): 285–90.

46. Wilson A, Zhou S, Bachoo P, et al. Systematic review of chimney and periscope grafts for endovascular aneurysm repair. Br J Surg 2013;100(12): 1557–64.

47. Donas KP, Torsello GB, Piccoli G, et al. The PROTAGORAS study to evaluate the performance of the Endurant stent graft for patients with pararenal pathologic processes treated by the chimney/snorkel endovascular technique. J Vasc Surg 2016; 63(1):1–7.

48. Donas KP, Lee JT, Lachat M, et al, Investigators OBOTP. Collected world experience about the

performance of the snorkel/chimney endovascular technique in the treatment of complex aortic pathologies: the PERICLES registry. Ann Surg 2015;262(3): 546–53.

49. Chaudhuri A, Dey R. Multi-component parallel endografts at complex TEVAR may be prone to modular dislocation causing novel endoleaks: a tale of two cases. EJVES Short Rep 2015;29:36–9.

50. Scali ST, Feezor RJ, Chang CK, et al. Critical analysis of results after chimney endovascular aortic aneurysm repair raises cause for concern. J Vasc Surg 2014;60(4):865–74.e1.

Treatment of Abdominal Aortic Pathology

Karol Meyermann, MD, Francis J. Caputo, MD*

KEYWORDS

- Abdominal aortic pathology • Endovascular repair • Abdominal aortic aneurysm • Treatment

KEY POINTS

- There are many treatment options for abdominal aortic pathology, particularly with the ever-expanding endovascular techniques.
- Surgical intervention is recommended when there is rapid aneurysmal expansion or the development of symptoms such as abdominal pain, tenderness, and back pain.
- Randomized, controlled studies and long-term results have shown better short- and medium-term outcomes when comparing endovascular aneurysm repair with open repair.
- Open aortic repair is increasingly being reserved for those with complex anatomy or a coexisting disease process that prohibits them from an endovascular repair.
- Current guidelines recommend endovascular repair for Trans-Atlantic Society Consensus (TASC) A disease and open repair for TASC D disease; there is an increasing trend for TASC B, C, and D lesions to be treated endovascularly.

INTRODUCTION

Abdominal aortic pathology is a diverse topic, ranging through a broad span of possible pathologies. The treatment options are equally vast, particularly with the ever-expanding endovascular techniques. In this article, we discuss management strategies for abdominal aortic aneurysms (AAA) and aortic occlusive disease, because they represent some of the most common pathologies encountered in clinical scenarios.

ANEURYSMAL DISEASE

Arterial aneurysms are defined as dilation greater than 1.5 times the expected arterial size.[1] In the abdominal aorta, the expected diameter is 2 cm; therefore, dilation greater than 3 cm is considered aneurysmal. Aortic aneurysms typically occur in the infrarenal aorta, but can occur anywhere along the vessel. The prevalence of AAA increases with age and is more common in men, occurring in 7% to 8% of men over 65 years of age.[2–5] Other etiologic factors include smoking, ethnic origin, family history, hypercholesterolemia, hypertension, and prior vascular disease.[6] Although aneurysms do increase with age, there are multiple processes that can contribute to aneurysm formation at younger ages, including inflammatory, infectious, genetic, and traumatic etiologies.

Indications for Elective Therapy

Surgical intervention is recommended when there is rapid aneurysmal expansion (>1 cm/y) or the development of symptoms such as abdominal pain, tenderness, and back pain, regardless of size. Such patients are at a higher risk of rupture as compared with asymptomatic patients or those with slower growth.[7,8] Treatment is also recommended when max diameter reaches 5.0 to 5.5 cm, owing to the relative risk of mortality associated with repair compared with aneurysm rupture.[9,10]

Division of Vascular Surgery, Department of Surgery, Cooper University Hospital, Suite 411, 3 Cooper Plaza, Camden, NJ 08103, USA
* Corresponding author.
E-mail address: Caputo-francis@cooperhealth.edu

Cardiol Clin 35 (2017) 431–439
http://dx.doi.org/10.1016/j.ccl.2017.03.009
0733-8651/17/© 2017 Elsevier Inc. All rights reserved.

cardiology.theclinics.com

Endovascular Treatment

Multiple, high-quality, randomized, controlled studies have shown better short- and medium-term outcomes when comparing endovascular aneurysm repair (EVAR) with open repair. Additionally, long-term results have been shown to be at least equivalent.[11-14] These data have driven EVAR to become the primary mode of therapy for the majority of patients with AAA. Open repair is generally preserved for patients with complex anatomy and is discussed elsewhere in this article.

With the advent of increasingly complex endovascular techniques and expanding indications for use, there has been an increase in use for such devices and both Medicare and the National Inpatient Sample have seen a decrease in the number of open aneurysm repairs performed.[11,12] There are a variety of endografts available on the market today and endovascular therapy represents approximately 70% of aortic aneurysm therapy provided today. New clinical trials and off label use of various devices has resulted in escalating innovation within endovascular therapy.

Although EVAR is an attractive option for an increasing number of patients, there are limitations to its use. The EVAR trial 1 and 2 (UK Endovascular Aneurysm Repair Trial 1 and 2) was a randomized control trial that looked at EVAR versus no intervention in high-risk patients with aneurysms greater than 5.5 cm. Although the 30-day mortality results were higher in the EVAR group, they demonstrated no difference between aneurysm-related or overall mortality between groups at 4 years. They also concluded that very high-risk patients do not benefit from AAA repair because they die from other causes before a benefit can be realized.[13,15] Despite this finding, many groups advocate for use of EVAR even in high-risk patients. Data from the VA National Surgical Quality Improvement Program showed that high-risk veterans undergoing EVAR showed a 30-day mortality rate of 3.4% and a 1-year mortality rate of 9.5% (**Table 1**).[16]

Postoperative complications

There are not a suitable amount of data to properly compare differences and complications between difference devices, given the wide variety and indications for use of different devices and the lack of long-term follow-up.

Endoleak An endoleak is defined as persistent blood flow within the aneurysm sac after EVAR. There are 5 recognized categories of endoleak, with distinct etiologies and treatment strategies.

- *Type I endoleak*: A type 1 endoleak describes blood flow from around either the proximal

Table 1
Results of major open versus EVAR trials

	Cardiac Morbidity (%)		All-Cause Mortality (%)	
	Open	EVAR	Open	EVAR
DREAM	5.7	5.3	4.6	1.2
OVER	—	—	4.7	1.7
EVAR-1	2.7	1.4	3.0	0.5

Abbreviations: DREAM, Dutch Randomized Endovascular Aneurysm Management; EVAR, endovascular aneurysm repair; OVER, Standard Open Surgery Versus Endovascular Repair of Abdominal Aortic Aneurysm.

(type 1a) or distal (type 1b) seal of the endograft. Type 1a endoleaks are typically treated in the operating room by deploying an extension or bare metal stent around the area of the leak. Type 1b endoleaks within the common iliac artery are treated by distal extension of the graft within the external iliac artery and occlusion of the hypogastric artery. When type 1 endoleaks are not responsive to traditional treatment strategies, an operative explant of the graft should be attempted owing to the high rate of rupture associated with type 1 endoleak.

- *Type 2 endoleak*: A type 2 endoleak is caused by backbleeding aortic branches into the aneurysm sac. The inferior mesenteric artery, lumbar arteries, or the middle sacral artery are responsible for such a leak. Of treated patients, 10% to 20% have evidence of type 2 endoleaks on postoperative computed tomography (CT) scans after EVAR.[17-20] Up to 80% of these leaks resolve within 12 months after EVAR.[21] Type 2 endoleaks are not treated unless there is enlargement of aneurysm sac size as because is a low likelihood of rupture with type 2 endoleaks.[20,22] Techniques to exclude type 2 endoleaks involve excluding the inflow and outflow vessels into the aneurysm sac.
- *Type 3 endoleak*: Type 3 endoleaks occur when there is destruction to the endograft's fabric or a leak between components of the graft. This can occur when there is stent graft fatigue in which the barbs or struts of the stent fracture under the continual mechanical stress during the cardiac cycle. Type 3 endoleaks occur in 0% to 1.5% of EVARs.[20,23] They can be successfully treated by relining the graft.
- *Type 4 endoleak*: Type 4 endoleaks are caused by porosity of the endograft. They

are less common in the current generation of devices. They typically resolve on their own once the aneurysm sac thromboses.

- *Type 5 endoleak*: Type 5 endoleaks are described as increased aneurysm sac pressure without a noticeable cause of endoleak; they are thus also described as "endotension." It is believed that the source is an undetected endoleak and they are initially treated with relining the endograft with proximal and distal extension.

Other complications of EVAR include graft migration, limb occlusion, neck dilation, stent infection, pelvic ischemia, or renal artery occlusion.

Follow-up

After EVAR, the Society for Vascular Surgery recommends that patients undergo CT scanning at 1 and 12 months in the first year after EVAR.[24] Granted there is also no evidence of endoleak or sac enlargement on the 12-month CT scan, patients can continue surveillance follow-up appointments using yearly duplex scans as the sole imaging modality (**Fig. 1**).[24,25]

Open Treatment

Open aortic repair is increasingly being reserved for those with complex anatomy or a coexisting disease process that prohibits them from undergoing an endovascular repair.[26–28] Anatomic constraints that mandate open repair include a hostile aortic neck, a narrow or calcified aortic bifurcation, iliac occlusive disease, infection of the aorta, or a prior aortic graft.[29] Although open repair is reserved for patients ineligible for EVAR, the current outcomes are continually improving, with perioperative mortality rates ranging from 1% to 7%.[30–32]

Preoperative assessment

Patients selected for open aortic intervention require an extensive workup before surgery. Owing the physiologic stress that occurs with cross-clamping the aorta, a comprehensive understanding of the patient's cardiac, pulmonary, and renal function is required.

Intraoperative management

Intraoperative management during open surgical repair of the abdominal aorta is a high-risk undertaking. The placement and removal an aortic cross-clamp results in a series of physiologic imbalances, which vary in accordance to where the clamp is placed.

- Cardiac function
  - Aortic clamping: During infraceliac clamping, blood flow is redirected to the splanchnic circulation, with little chance in preload owing to the high venous capacity of the splanchnic circulation. During supraceliac clamping of the aorta, there is a huge increase in preload and afterload. Left

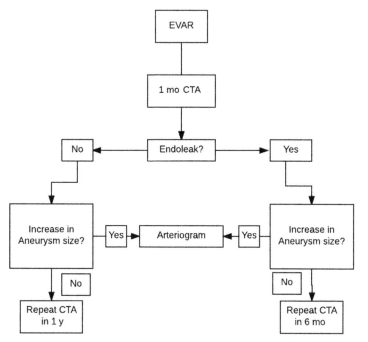

Fig. 1. Surveillance after endovascular aneurysm repair (EVAR). CTA, computed tomography angiography.

ventricular wall abnormalities were noted in 92% of patients with supraceliac cross-clamps, as compared with 33% of patients with suprarenal cross-clamps and none of patients with infrarenal cross-clamps.[33]

○ Aortic declamping: There is a dramatic decrease in arterial pressure owing to the instant reduction in peripheral vascular resistance after unclamping the aorta. As blood flow is returned to ischemic tissue, the reperfusion hyperemia results in further central hypotension. Toxic metabolites, lactic acid, reactive oxygen species, and prostaglandins that accumulated within ischemia tissue during the aortic cross-clamp time are now returned to circulation, promoting vasodilation and myocardial depression.

- Renal function: Renal flow is compromised even with the placement of the aortic clamp infrarenally; renal blood flow during infrarenal clamp placement decreases by up to 40%.[34,35] The increase in renal vascular resistance and decrease in the glomerular filtration rate can continue for up to 60 minutes after the clamp is removed.[35] Although various pharmacological agents have been suggested to provide renal protection during aortic cross-clamping, there is no clinical evidence that such interventions are successful.[36–39] Renal hypothermia has been reported by many groups to improve renal outcomes after suprarenal aortic clamping.[40–44]

Postoperative complications

Complications after open aneurysm repair are relatively common, occurring in up to 76% of patients.[45]

Early complications

- Bleeding: If there is a persistent need for transfusion, volume resuscitation, or vasoactive medications to maintain adequate blood pressure, bleeding complications should be considered.[46]
- Myocardial infarction: Myocardial infarction occurs in up to 10% of patients in the perioperative period.[46]
- Respiratory failure: Respiratory complications are the most common complication after open aneurysm repair, with 17% of patients developing postoperative pneumonia.[46] Respiratory complications in any form are associated with decreased long-term survival.[47]
- Renal failure: Postoperative renal insufficiency occurs in 15% to 20% of patients who undergo an open juxtarenal aneurysm repair,

but only 3.5% of patients required renal replacement therapy.[48]

- Colonic ischemia: There is a clinical incidence of 0.2% to 6% after open aneurysm repair.[45,49–52]
- Spinal cord ischemia: Although spinal cord ischemia is a rare events, occurring in less than 1% of all open repairs, it is significant in that it correlates with poor functional outcomes and significantly reduced survival.[47,53,54]
- Venous thrombosis: Pulmonary embolism is uncommon, occurring at a rate of 1.4%.[55]

Late complications Late complications related to open aneurysm repair are rare, with 10-year event-free survival rates ranging from 91% to 95%.[56,57] Long-term complications are known to occur and include anastomotic pseudoaneurysms, graft infection, and abdominal wall hernias.

Follow-up and surveillance

Patients undergoing open aneurysm repair require less frequent follow-up than patients having an endovascular repair. Society for Vascular Surgery guidelines recommend surveillance imaging with duplex once at least every 5 years or more often if there is a cause for concern.[24]

Ruptures

Approximately only 25% of patients with a ruptured AAA make it to the hospital alive.[7] Transfer to high-volume regional centers can significantly lower the mortality for ruptured AAA patients.[58] Most ruptured AAA patients (>70%) undergo EVAR; multiple trials have shown the benefit of pursuing endovascular over open repair when feasible.[14,59]

Resuscitation once patients have arrived at the hospital should aim toward limiting the administration of intravenous fluids, because the resultant increase in blood pressure may overcome the tamponade that is currently stabilizing their rupture. Aggressive volume resuscitation during the initial management of ruptured AAA before proximal aortic control is a predictor of increased postoperative mortality (**Fig. 2**).[60]

The decision to pursue an open versus endovascular approach once the diagnosis has been made depends on patient anatomy and facilities available. Two metaanalyses determined that 47% to 67% of patients with ruptured AAA have anatomy suitable to EVAR with current devices.[61,62] Patients with ruptured AAA tend to have larger infrarenal aortic diameters and shorter neck lengths than patients with nonruptured AAA.[63,64] A recent review looked at the outcomes of hostile neck anatomy on patients undergoing

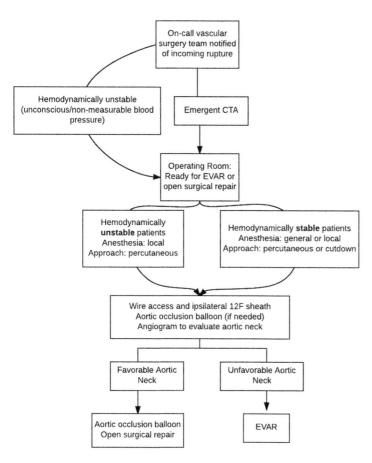

Fig. 2. The Albany Vascular Group standardized protocol for ruptured aortic repair. CTA, computed tomography angiography; EVAR, endovascular aneurysm repair.

EVAR. They found that only 34% of patients with ruptured AAA had neck morphology that would meet the indication for use for available stent-grafts.

Predictors of Mortality

Factors associated with a reduction in survival after open repair of ruptured AAA include loss of consciousness, preoperative cardiac arrest, preexisting congestive heart failure, preexisting renal insufficiency, advanced age, female gender, nonwhite race, and APACHE II (Acute Physiologic and Chronic Health Evaluation) score.[52,65–68]

OCCLUSIVE DISEASE

Occlusive disease of the distal aorta and iliac arteries typically presents as buttock and thigh claudication, because exertional muscle fatigue commonly presents 1 level below the level of disease. Determination of treatment type varies in accordance to the extent of disease. The Trans-Atlantic Society Consensus (TASC) Classification divides lesions into A, B, C, or D according to

length and morphology and has guidelines for treatment between classifications.

The Inter-Society Consensus for the Management of Peripheral Arterial Disease currently recommends endovascular repair for TASC A disease and open repair for TASC D disease. TASC B/C lesions are up to the discretion of the surgeon and informed consent of the patient.[69] However, there is an increasing trend for TASC B, C, and D lesions to be treated endovascularly.

Evaluation

Evaluation of suspected aortoiliac occlusive disease can be done with noninvasive studies, such as segmental systolic blood pressure measurements and pulse volume recordings. In patients with clinical and noninvasive findings suggestive of aortoiliac disease, CT angiography should be obtained to determine the extent of disease.

Medical Therapy

Optimal medical therapy should be recommended for all patients with symptoms of lower extremity peripheral arterial disease, even when they clearly also require surgical intervention.

Endovascular Treatment

Indications for intervention in aortoiliac occlusive disease include disabling claudication, ischemic rest pain, or tissue loss. According to the TASC II recommendations, technical and clinical success of percutaneous transluminal angioplasty in iliac stenosis is greater than 90% with technical success in recanalization long segment iliac occlusions to be around 80% to 85%.[69] The use of endovascular aortoiliac interventions have surged in popularity since their introduction and are in use for increasingly complex anatomy. Endovascular aortoiliac interventions have increased by 850% between 1995 and 2000 in a National Inpatient Sample while aortobifemoral bypass surgery decreased by 16% during the same time period. Although earlier studies reported lower patency rates for TASC C and D lesions, more recent studies have reported patency rates on par with open intervention.[70]

The STAG trial (Randomized Clinical Trial of Stents Versus Angioplasty for the Treatment of Iliac Artery Occlusions) was a randomized trial for management of iliac artery occlusion that looked at percutaneous transluminal angioplasty versus primary stenting. It was stopped early owing to significantly higher rates of complications within the percutaneous transluminal angioplasty group, primarily owing to embolic phenomena. There were also higher rates of technical success within the primary stenting group.[71]

The COBEST trial (Covered versus Balloon Expandable Stent Trial) was a prospective multicenter, randomized trial looking at covered versus bare metal stents in aortoiliac disease. Covered stents significantly reduced restenosis, but this finding was only present in TASC C/D lesions. The odds ratio for 18-month restenosis also favored covered stents in a variety of subgroup analyses, most prominently in males and smokers.[72]

Open Surgical Treatment

Severe aortoiliac occlusive disease, such as TASC C and D lesions, is typically treated using a variety of open surgical approaches, including aortobifemoral bypass, aortoiliac endarterectomy, iliofemoral bypass, or extra-anatomic bypass. Open surgical repair is believed to have higher patency rates than endovascular therapy for high grade lesions.[73] However, a single center review at the Cleveland Clinic demonstrated that, although rates of primary patency were significantly better in the open surgery patients, rates of secondary patency, limb salvage, and overall survival were not significantly different.

Aortobifemoral bypass is considered to be the gold standard treatment for hemodynamically significant aortobiiliac disease in low-risk patients given its safety and efficacy (mortality rate <5%; 5-year patency rates >80%).

Extra-anatomic bypass grafts are an alternative form of revascularization in patients who are high risk with multiple medical comorbidities, have had multiple prior abdominal procedures, multiple adhesions, or previous pelvic irradiation, have intraabdominal sepsis, or have failed endovascular therapy.

Complications

Morbidity after aortic surgery for occlusive disease ranges from 17% to 32%, with cardiac complications being most common cause of mortality.[74] Pulmonary complications are also common and are most likely to occur in the elderly or those with chronic obstructive pulmonary disease or smokers.[75] Pain control, appropriate diuresis, and pulmonary toilet are important measures to prevent respiratory complications. Late complications after aortobifemoral bypass include graft limb thrombosis, aortoenteric fistula, graft infection, and anastomotic pseudoaneurysm.

SUMMARY

The treatment of aortic pathology is an evolving field with advances in endovascular and open aortic options that are continually undergoing advancement.

REFERENCES

1. Johnston KW, Rutherford RB, Tilson MD, et al. Suggested standards for reporting on arterial aneurysms. Subcommittee on Reporting Standards for Arterial Aneurysms, Ad Hoc Committee on Reporting Standards, Society for Vascular Surgery and North American Chapter, International Society for Cardiovascular Surgery. J Vasc Surg 1991;13(3): 452–8.
2. Ashton HA, Buxton MJ, Day NE, et al. The Multicentre Aneurysm Screening Study (MASS) into the effect of abdominal aortic aneurysm screening on mortality in men: a randomised controlled trial. Lancet 2002;360(9345):1531–9.
3. Lucarotti M, Shaw E, Poskitt K, et al. The Gloucestershire Aneurysm Screening Programme: the first 2 years' experience. Eur J Vasc Surg 1993;7(4): 397–401.
4. Vardulaki KA, Walker NM, Day NE, et al. Quantifying the risks of hypertension, age, sex and smoking in

patients with abdominal aortic aneurysm. Br J Surg 2000;87(2):195–200.

5. Norman PE, Jamrozik K, Lawrence-Brown MM, et al. Population based randomised controlled trial on impact of screening on mortality from abdominal aortic aneurysm. BMJ 2004;329(7477):1259.

6. Lederle FA, Johnson GR, Wilson SE, et al. Prevalence and associations of abdominal aortic aneurysm detected through screening. Aneurysm Detection and Management (ADAM) Veterans Affairs Cooperative Study Group. Ann Intern Med 1997;126(6):441–9.

7. Mortality results for randomised controlled trial of early elective surgery or ultrasonographic surveillance for small abdominal aortic aneurysms. The UK Small Aneurysm Trial Participants. Lancet 1998;352(9141):1649–55.

8. Lederle FA, Wilson SE, Johnson GR, et al. Design of the abdominal aortic aneurysm detection and management study. ADAM VA Cooperative study group. J Vasc Surg 1994;20(2):296–303.

9. Chaikof EL, Brewster DC, Dalman RL, et al. The care of patients with an abdominal aortic aneurysm: the Society for Vascular Surgery practice guidelines. J Vasc Surg 2009;50(4 Suppl):S2–49.

10. Moll FL, Powell JT, Fraedrich G, et al. Management of abdominal aortic aneurysms clinical practice guidelines of the European society for vascular surgery. Eur J Vasc Endovasc Surg 2011;41(Suppl 1):S1–58.

11. De Bruin JL, Baas AF, Buth J, et al. Long-term outcome of open or endovascular repair of abdominal aortic aneurysm. N Engl J Med 2010;362(20):1881–9.

12. Becquemin JP, Pillet JC, Lescalie F, et al. A randomized controlled trial of endovascular aneurysm repair versus open surgery for abdominal aortic aneurysms in low- to moderate-risk patients. J Vasc Surg 2011;53(5):1167–73.e1161.

13. Greenhalgh RM, Brown LC, Kwong GP, et al, EVAR Trial Participants. Comparison of endovascular aneurysm repair with open repair in patients with abdominal aortic aneurysm (EVAR trial 1), 30-day operative mortality results: randomised controlled trial. Lancet 2004;364(9437):843–8.

14. Lederle FA, Freischlag JA, Kyriakides TC, et al. Long-term comparison of endovascular and open repair of abdominal aortic aneurysm. N Engl J Med 2012;367(21):1988–97.

15. EVAR Trial Participants. Endovascular aneurysm repair and outcome in patients unfit for open repair of abdominal aortic aneurysm (EVAR trial 2): randomised controlled trial. Lancet 2005;365(9478):2187–92.

16. Bush RL, Johnson ML, Hedayati N, et al. Performance of endovascular aortic aneurysm repair in high-risk patients: results from the Veterans Affairs National Surgical Quality Improvement Program. J Vasc Surg 2007;45(2):227–33 [discussion: 233–5].

17. Chuter TA, Faruqi RM, Sawhney R, et al. Endoleak after endovascular repair of abdominal aortic aneurysm. J Vasc Surg 2001;34(1):98–105.

18. Buth J, Harris PL, van Marrewijk C, et al. The significance and management of different types of endoleaks. Semin Vasc Surg 2003;16(2):95–102.

19. Sheehan MK, Ouriel K, Greenberg R, et al. Are type II endoleaks after endovascular aneurysm repair endograft dependent? J Vasc Surg 2006;43(4):657–61.

20. van Marrewijk C, Buth J, Harris PL, et al. Significance of endoleaks after endovascular repair of abdominal aortic aneurysms: the EUROSTAR experience. J Vasc Surg 2002;35(3):461–73.

21. Brewster DC, Jones JE, Chung TK, et al. Long-term outcomes after endovascular abdominal aortic aneurysm repair: the first decade. Ann Surg 2006;244(3):426–38.

22. Karthikesalingam A, Thrumurthy SG, Jackson D, et al. Current evidence is insufficient to define an optimal threshold for intervention in isolated type II endoleak after endovascular aneurysm repair. J Endovasc Ther 2012;19(2):200–8.

23. Sandford RM, Bown MJ, Fishwick G, et al. Duplex ultrasound scanning is reliable in the detection of endoleak following endovascular aneurysm repair. Eur J Vasc Endovasc Surg 2006;32(5):537–41.

24. Chaikof EL, Brewster DC, Dalman RL, et al. SVS practice guidelines for the care of patients with an abdominal aortic aneurysm: executive summary. J Vasc Surg 2009;50(4):880–96.

25. Sternbergh WC 3rd, Greenberg RK, Chuter TA, et al. Redefining postoperative surveillance after endovascular aneurysm repair: recommendations based on 5-year follow-up in the US Zenith multicenter trial. J Vasc Surg 2008;48(2):278–84 [discussion: 284–5].

26. Albuquerque FC Jr, Tonnessen BH, Noll RE Jr, et al. Paradigm shifts in the treatment of abdominal aortic aneurysm: trends in 721 patients between 1996 and 2008. J Vasc Surg 2010;51(6):1348–52 [discussion: 1352–3].

27. Costin JA, Watson DR, Duff SB, et al. Evaluation of the complexity of open abdominal aneurysm repair in the era of endovascular stent grafting. J Vasc Surg 2006;43(5):915–20.

28. Joels CS, Langan EM 3rd, Daley CA, et al. Changing indications and outcomes for open abdominal aortic aneurysm repair since the advent of endovascular repair. Am Surg 2009;75(8):665–9 [discussion: 669–70].

29. Moise MA, Woo EY, Velazquez OC, et al. Barriers to endovascular aortic aneurysm repair: past experience and implications for future device development. Vasc Endovascular Surg 2006;40(3):197–203.

30. Lee HG, Clair DG, Ouriel K. Ten-year comparison of all-cause mortality after endovascular or open repair of abdominal aortic aneurysms: a propensity score analysis. World J Surg 2013;37(3):680–7.

31. Landon BE, O'Malley AJ, Giles K, et al. Volume-outcome relationships and abdominal aortic aneurysm repair. Circulation 2010;122(13):1290–7.

32. Martin MC, Giles KA, Pomposelli FB, et al. National outcomes after open repair of abdominal aortic aneurysms with visceral or renal bypass. Ann Vasc Surg 2010;24(1):106–12.

33. Roizen MF, Beaupre PN, Alpert RA, et al. Monitoring with two-dimensional transesophageal echocardiography. Comparison of myocardial function in patients undergoing supraceliac, suprarenal-infraceliac, or infrarenal aortic occlusion. J Vasc Surg 1984;1(2):300–5.

34. Gamulin Z, Forster A, Morel D, et al. Effects of infrarenal aortic cross-clamping on renal hemodynamics in humans. Anesthesiology 1984;61(4):394–9.

35. Abbott WM, Austen WG. The reversal of renal cortical ischemia during aortic occlusion by mannitol. J Surg Res 1974;16(5):482–9.

36. Schoenwald PK. Intraoperative management of renal function in the surgical patient at risk. Focus on aortic surgery. Anesthesiol Clin North America 2000;18(4):719–37.

37. Macedo E, Abdulkader R, Castro I, et al. Lack of protection of N-acetylcysteine (NAC) in acute renal failure related to elective aortic aneurysm repair-a randomized controlled trial. Nephrol Dial Transplant 2006;21(7):1863–9.

38. Hynninen MS, Niemi TT, Poyhia R, et al. N-acetylcysteine for the prevention of kidney injury in abdominal aortic surgery: a randomized, double-blind, placebo-controlled trial. Anesth Analg 2006;102(6):1638–45.

39. Hersey P, Poullis M. Does the administration of mannitol prevent renal failure in open abdominal aortic aneurysm surgery? Interact Cardiovasc Thorac Surg 2008;7(5):906–9.

40. Patel VI, Ergul E, Conrad MF, et al. Continued favorable results with open surgical repair of type IV thoracoabdominal aortic aneurysms. J Vasc Surg 2011;53(6):1492–8.

41. Ochsner JL, Mills NL, Gardner PA. A technique for renal preservation during suprarenal abdominal aortic operations. Surg Gynecol Obstet 1984;159(4):388–90.

42. Schmitto JD, Fatehpur S, Tezval H, et al. Hypothermic renal protection using cold histidine-tryptophan-ketoglutarate solution perfusion in suprarenal aortic surgery. Ann Vasc Surg 2008;22(4):520–4.

43. Tsai S, Conrad MF, Patel VI, et al. Durability of open repair of juxtarenal abdominal aortic aneurysms. J Vasc Surg 2012;56(1):2–7.

44. Yeung KK, Jongkind V, Coveliers HM, et al. Routine continuous cold perfusion of the kidneys during elective juxtarenal aortic aneurysm repair. Eur J Vasc Endovasc Surg 2008;35(4):446–51.

45. Zwolak RM, Sidawy AN, Greenberg RK, et al. Lifeline registry of endovascular aneurysm repair: open repair surgical controls in clinical trials. J Vasc Surg 2008;48(3):511–8.

46. Schermerhorn ML, O'Malley AJ, Jhaveri A, et al. Endovascular vs. open repair of abdominal aortic aneurysms in the Medicare population. N Engl J Med 2008;358(5):464–74.

47. Nathan DP, Brinster CJ, Jackson BM, et al. Predictors of decreased short- and long-term survival following open abdominal aortic aneurysm repair. J Vasc Surg 2011;54(5):1237–43.

48. Tallarita T, Sobreira ML, Oderich GS. Results of open pararenal abdominal aortic aneurysm repair: tabular review of the literature. Ann Vasc Surg 2011;25(1):143–9.

49. Bjorck M, Troeng T, Bergqvist D. Risk factors for intestinal ischaemia after aortoiliac surgery: a combined cohort and case-control study of 2824 operations. Eur J Vasc Endovasc Surg 1997;13(6):531–9.

50. Brewster DC, Franklin DP, Cambria RP, et al. Intestinal ischemia complicating abdominal aortic surgery. Surgery 1991;109(4):447–54.

51. Longo WE, Lee TC, Barnett MG, et al. Ischemic colitis complicating abdominal aortic aneurysm surgery in the U.S. veteran. J Surg Res 1996;60(2):351–4.

52. Becquemin JP, Majewski M, Fermani N, et al. Colon ischemia following abdominal aortic aneurysm repair in the era of endovascular abdominal aortic repair. J Vasc Surg 2008;47(2):258–63 [discussion: 263].

53. Crawford RS, Pedraza JD, Chung TK, et al. Functional outcome after thoracoabdominal aneurysm repair. J Vasc Surg 2008;48(4):828–35.

54. Patel VI, Lancaster RT, Conrad MF, et al. Comparable mortality with open repair of complex and infrarenal aortic aneurysm. J Vasc Surg 2011;54(4):952–9.

55. de Maistre E, Terriat B, Lesne-Padieu AS, et al. High incidence of venous thrombosis after surgery for abdominal aortic aneurysm. J Vasc Surg 2009;49(3):596–601.

56. Conrad MF, Crawford RS, Pedraza JD, et al. Long-term durability of open abdominal aortic aneurysm repair. J Vasc Surg 2007;46(4):669–75.

57. Adam DJ, Fitridge RA, Raptis S. Late reintervention for aortic graft-related events and new aortoiliac disease after open abdominal aortic aneurysm repair in an Australian population. J Vasc Surg 2006;43(4):701–5 [discussion: 705–6].

58. Holt PJ, Poloniecki JD, Gerrard D, et al. Meta-analysis and systematic review of the relationship

between volume and outcome in abdominal aortic aneurysm surgery. Br J Surg 2007;94(4):395–403.

59. Prinssen M, Verhoeven EL, Buth J, et al. A randomized trial comparing conventional and endovascular repair of abdominal aortic aneurysms. N Engl J Med 2004;351(16):1607–18.

60. Dick F, Erdoes G, Opfermann P, et al. Delayed volume resuscitation during initial management of ruptured abdominal aortic aneurysm. J Vasc Surg 2013;57(4):943–50.

61. Mastracci TM, Garrido-Olivares L, Cina CS, et al. Endovascular repair of ruptured abdominal aortic aneurysms: a systematic review and meta-analysis. J Vasc Surg 2008;47(1):214–21.

62. Harkin DW, Dillon M, Blair PH, et al. Endovascular ruptured abdominal aortic aneurysm repair (EV-RAR): a systematic review. Eur J Vasc Endovasc Surg 2007;34(6):673–81.

63. Hinchliffe RJ, Alric P, Rose D, et al. Comparison of morphologic features of intact and ruptured aneurysms of infrarenal abdominal aorta. J Vasc Surg 2003;38(1):88–92.

64. Badger SA, O'Donnell ME, Makar RR, et al. Aortic necks of ruptured abdominal aneurysms dilate more than asymptomatic aneurysms after endovascular repair. J Vasc Surg 2006;44(2):244–9.

65. Bauer EP, Redaelli C, von Segesser LK, et al. Ruptured abdominal aortic aneurysms: predictors for early complications and death. Surgery 1993; 114(1):31–5.

66. Noel AA, Gloviczki P, Cherry KJ Jr, et al. Ruptured abdominal aortic aneurysms: the excessive mortality rate of conventional repair. J Vasc Surg 2001;34(1): 41–6.

67. Piper G, Patel NA, Chandela S, et al. Short-term predictors and long-term outcome after ruptured abdominal aortic aneurysm repair. Am Surg 2003; 69(8):703–9 [discussion: 709–10].

68. Gloviczki P, Pairolero PC, Mucha P Jr, et al. Ruptured abdominal aortic aneurysms: repair should not be denied. J Vasc Surg 1992;15(5):851–7 [discussion: 857–9].

69. Norgren L, Hiatt WR, Dormandy JA, et al. Inter-Society Consensus for the management of peripheral arterial disease (TASC II). J Vasc Surg 2007; 45(Suppl S):S5–67.

70. Kashyap VS, Pavkov ML, Bena JF, et al. The management of severe aortoiliac occlusive disease: endovascular therapy rivals open reconstruction. J Vasc Surg 2008;48(6):1451–7, 1457.e1–3.

71. Goode SD, Cleveland TJ, Gaines PA, STAG Trial Collaborators. Randomized clinical trial of stents versus angioplasty for the treatment of iliac artery occlusions (STAG trial). Br J Surg 2013;100(9):1148–53.

72. Mwipatayi BP, Sharma S, Daneshmand A, et al. Durability of the balloon-expandable covered versus bare-metal stents in the Covered versus Balloon Expandable Stent Trial (COBEST) for the treatment of aortoiliac occlusive disease. J Vasc Surg 2016; 64(1):83–94.e81.

73. Hans SS, DeSantis D, Siddiqui R, et al. Results of endovascular therapy and aortobifemoral grafting for Transatlantic Inter-Society type C and D aortoiliac occlusive disease. Surgery 2008;144(4):583–9 [discussion: 589–90].

74. Martinez BD, Hertzer NR, Beven EG. Influence of distal arterial occlusive disease on prognosis following aortobifemoral bypass. Surgery 1980; 88(6):795–805.

75. Garibaldi RA, Britt MR, Coleman ML, et al. Risk factors for postoperative pneumonia. Am J Med 1981; 70(3):677–80.

Blunt Trauma of the Aorta, Current Guidelines

Marc D. Trust, MD, Pedro G.R. Teixeira, MD*

KEYWORDS

- Blunt injury • Thoracic aorta • Aortic transection • Pseudoaneurysm • Endovascular repair • TEVAR
- Diagnosis • Management

KEY POINTS

- Computed tomography scanning is the imaging modality of choice for blunt thoracic aortic injury (BTAI) diagnosis and repair planning.
- Endovascular repair of BTAI is associated with improved survival and has become the standard of care.
- With institution of strict blood pressure control, in-hospital rupture of BTAI is reduced and delayed repair is possible, with improved survival.

HISTORY

In 1557, Andreas Vesalius reported the first case of blunt thoracic aortic injury (BTAI).[1] Understanding of this injury was further advanced by Parmley and colleagues[2] in 1958 with their landmark publication describing 296 cases of BTAI with detailed autopsy and clinical information. After the first successful repair of this injury by Klassen (as reported by Passaro),[3] open repair became the primary treatment modality for blunt thoracic aortic injuries. With the advent of endografts and the remarkable evolution of endovascular techniques and reports of improved outcomes with its use for degenerative disease of the aorta, their application in the traumatic setting followed suit, and in 1997, Kato and colleagues[4] reported the first use of these devices to repair a traumatic injury using an endovascular technique. This paradigm shift in the management of traumatic thoracic aortic injuries was quickly embraced by the surgical community and improved survival was widely demonstrated with the endovascular approach.[5] Endovascular repair has now replaced open techniques as the primary treatment modality for BTAI and became the standard of care. These changing paradigms in all aspects of care of this injury are discussed in this article.

EPIDEMIOLOGY

BTAI is the second leading cause of mortality in trauma patients.[6] A previous National Trauma Data Bank study reported an overall incidence of 0.3% of all trauma admissions over a 6-year study period.[7] According to a 2008 multicenter American Association for the Surgery of Trauma (AAST) study including 196 patients, 68% were the result of motor vehicle collision, 13% from motorcycle collisions, 7% from falls, and 6% from auto–pedestrian accidents, and 6% from other mechanisms.[8] Autopsy studies have placed the prehospital mortality rates of this injury at 57% to 80%, and showed that more than one-third of patients who survived to hospital presentation died within 4 hours.[9,10] Furthermore, these studies also showed substantial mortality associated with other injuries such as brain, cardiac,

Disclosure Statement: The authors have nothing to disclose.
Conflict of Interest: None.
Department of Surgery and Perioperative Care, Dell Medical School, University of Texas at Austin, 1501 Red River Street, Austin, TX 78712, USA
* Corresponding author. University Medical Center Brackenridge, 601 East 15th Street, Austin, TX 78701.
E-mail address: pgteixeira@seton.org

Cardiol Clin 35 (2017) 441–451
http://dx.doi.org/10.1016/j.ccl.2017.03.010
0733-8651/17/© 2017 Elsevier Inc. All rights reserved.

hemothorax, intraabdominal, and pulmonary injuries as well as rib and lower extremity fractures. Overall survival in patients who do not suffer early mortality is good. Earlier rates reported in the literature range from 13% to 19%.[7,8] Recently, another AAST-sponsored multicenter study including 382 patients reported an overall mortality rate of 18.8%; however, the aortic-related mortality was reported at only 6.5%.[11]

DIAGNOSIS

With the widespread adoption of Advanced Trauma Life Support principles, the majority of trauma patients are receiving a chest radiograph as a part of their initial workup. This tool has been the primary screening modality used for BTAI. Many radiographic features have been described as being associated with aortic injury, most commonly a widened mediastinum (**Fig. 1**). Other findings include obliteration of aortic contour, loss of paravertebral pleural stripe, displacement of left mainstem bronchus, deviation of the nasogastric tube, and left apical cap (**Box 1**).[1] Several studies have assessed the usefulness of the chest radiograph as a screening tool for BTAI. Ekeh and colleagues[12] published their findings in which patients with BTAI were found to have abnormal chest radiograph findings 89% of the time. This was compared with a control group of patients without BTAI, in which only 50% of patients were thought to have abnormal findings that warranted further studies More recently, Gutierrez and colleagues[13] published their retrospective findings in which a total of 17 patients with BTAI were identified over a 3-year period. Of these, only 7 (41%) had positive chest radiograph findings; however, of these 7 patients 95% were

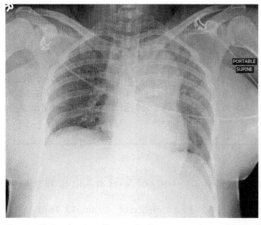

Fig. 1. Plain chest radiograph demonstrating widened mediastinum.

Box 1
Possible chest radiograph findings in patients with blunt thoracic aortic injury
Wide mediastinum (supine chest radiograph >8 cm; upright chest radiograph >6 cm)
Obscured, indistinct or enlarged aortic knob; abnormal aortic arch contour
Left apical cap (extrapleural apical hematoma)
Large left hemothorax
Deviation of nasogastric tube to the right
Deviation of trachea rightward
Downward displacement of the left mainstem bronchus
Upward displacement of the right mainstem bronchus
Wide left paravertebral stripe

confirmed to have an injury on computed tomography (CT) imaging.

Because of the significant number of patients who present with an initial normal chest radiograph despite having a BTAI, this imaging modality cannot be considered an adequate screening tool for this injury. A high level of suspicion for a BTAI should be present for all patients injured in a high-energy mechanism. In those instances, liberal use of chest CT is warranted and should be the primary screening and diagnostic imaging modality. In fact, CT scan has vastly replaced conventional angiography as the gold standard test for diagnosis of BTAI. Findings of 2 separate AAST studies, the first of which completed in 1997 and the second in 2007, showed a dramatic increase in CT use and elimination of conventional angiography for diagnostic purposes. In the initial study, 87% of patients underwent aortography, compared with only 8% of patients in the second, and the use of CT scan increased from 35% to 93%[5] Furthermore, current CT scanners have been shown to achieve 100% sensitivity and specificity for BTAI.[1] Recent evidence-based guidelines published by the Eastern Association for the Surgery of Trauma in 2015 recommend that patients suspected of having a BTAI undergo CT scanning of the chest over aortography, because it is more readily available, less invasive, less time consuming, and allows for the identification of other associated thoracic injuries that are commonly present (**Fig. 2**).[6] The CT scan has the added benefits of not only providing detailed information about the aortic anatomy (**Fig. 3**) and fully assess the severity of the aortic injury (**Figs. 4** and **5**), but also depicting aberrant

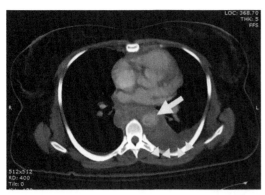

Fig. 2. Chest computed tomography scan, axial view, demonstrating proximal descending thoracic aorta pseudoaneurysm (*arrow*) with associated moderate left hemothorax (*arrowheads*).

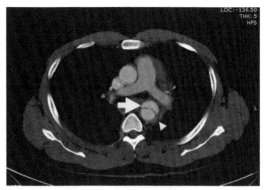

Fig. 4. Chest computed tomography scan, axial view. Proximal descending thoracic aorta pseudoaneurysm (*arrow*). Small periaortic hematoma (*arrowhead*).

anatomy (**Figs. 6** and **7**) and serving as an important tool for preprocedural planning for endovascular repair (**Fig. 8**).

The most widely used grading system is the one put forth by the Society for Vascular Surgery (SVS) and injury grades range from minor partial thickness injury to complete transection. Injuries confined to the intima are classified as grade I. When intramural hematomas or larger intimal flaps are present, the injuries progress to grade II. Grade III injuries are characterized by the presence of a pseudoaneurysm in which only the adventitia remains intact, and a complete transection or rupture is classified as a grade IV injury (**Table 1**).[14] Recently, data from Harborview Medical Center has been published suggesting a more simplified grading system placing injuries into categories of mild, moderate, or severe. In this system, mild

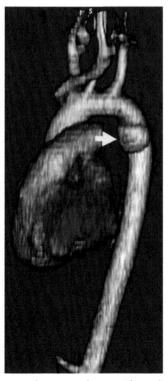

Fig. 3. Computed tomography scan. Three-dimensional reconstruction demonstrating proximal descending thoracic aorta pseudoaneurysm (*arrow*).

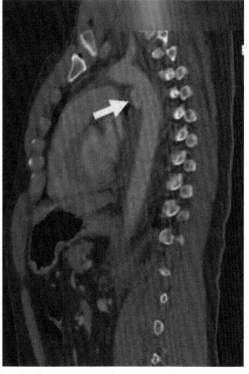

Fig. 5. Chest computed tomography scan, sagittal view. Proximal descending thoracic pseudoaneurysm (*arrow*).

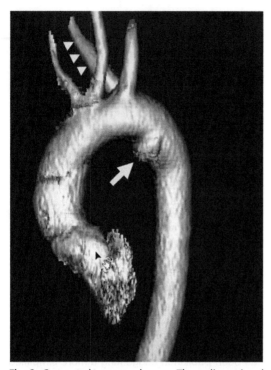

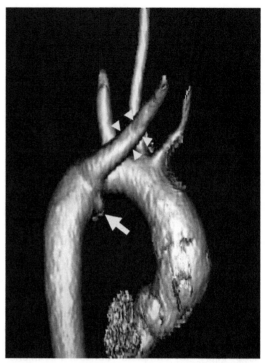

Fig. 6. Computed tomography scan. Three-dimensional reconstruction demonstrating proximal descending thoracic aorta pseudoaneurysm (*arrow*) and aberrant right subclavian artery (*arrowheads*) originating from the posterior aspect of the descending thoracic aorta, distal to the origin of the left subclavian artery.

Fig. 7. Computed tomography scan. Three-dimensional reconstruction (posterior view) demonstrating proximal descending thoracic aorta pseudoaneurysm (*arrow*) and aberrant right subclavian artery (*arrowheads*) originating from the posterior aspect of the descending thoracic aorta, distal to the origin of the left subclavian artery.

injuries are those with no external contour abnormality or an intimal tear of less than 10 mm; moderate includes injuries showing external contour, such as pseudoaneurysm or an intimal tear of greater than 10 mm; and severe injuries have active extravasation of contrast or contained rupture with a left subclavian hematoma of greater than 15 mm in size.[15] Current evidence-based treatment guidelines depend on injury grades, which are discussed in the next section.

MANAGEMENT

Previously, once the diagnosis of BTAI was made, management proceeded immediately with thoracotomy for open repair to minimize the risk of aortic rupture. Starting in the 1980s, evidence for the use of antihypertensive medications to decrease the risk of rupture and safety of delay in intervention began to emerge.[16–19] In 1998, Fabian and the group in Memphis published one of the first prospective studies evaluating the use of antihypertensive medications, and reported that no patients suffered in-hospital rupture when managed in this manner as either a bridge

to delayed repair or as a primary treatment modality.[16] Currently, once the diagnosis is made, antihypertensives are started as early as tolerated and systolic blood pressure is maintained to a goal of 90 to 120 mm Hg.[6,20] At our institution, all patients with BTAI are admitted to the intensive care unit and invasive blood pressure monitoring is used. Patients are first started on an esmolol drip to achieve the aforementioned blood pressure parameters. A second antihypertensive drip such as nicardipine is used if blood pressure parameters cannot be met with esmolol alone.

Once initial management with antihypertensive medications is initiated, the decision of definitive management must be made. The 2011 guidelines set forth by the SVS suggest that although grade I injuries may be managed nonoperatively, grades II through IV injuries should be repaired. These recommendations are based on their systematic review of the available literature at the time of publication that showed a mortality rate of approximately 46% in patients treated nonoperatively.[14] More recently, the previously mentioned study by Heneghan and colleagues,[15] which called for a more simplified grading system reported that no

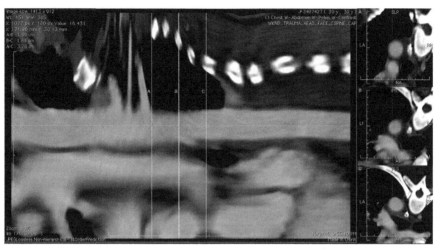

Fig. 8. Computed tomography scan imaging manipulation using commercially available software demonstrating center line utilization for endovascular repair planning.

patients with minimal grade injuries who had follow-up imaging (n = 38) showed progression of the injury. They concluded that patients with these minimal injures can be managed nonoperatively, with optional surveillance imaging, whereas moderate and severe injuries required definitive therapy.

Recently, several studies have been published suggesting that not all injuries containing a pseudoaneurysm must be repaired. Rabin and colleagues reported in their single institution retrospective review of 97 patients that 46% of patients were managed without intervention, and none of these suffered aortic-related mortality, complications, or required emergent interventions. Furthermore, 31 patients had follow-up for an average of 3.8 months, and only 1 showed progression of injury to warrant repair. This nonoperative group included injuries with intimal tears and pseudoaneurysm of various sizes. The authors also suggest that secondary signs of injury, such as pseudocoarctation, mediastinal hematoma with mass effect, or large left hemothorax, are indicators of a higher risk of rupture warranting urgent repair. They concluded that injuries with a pseudoaneurysm smaller than 50% of the circumference of the aorta are amendable to nonoperative management. Harris and colleagues[21] from the same group in Baltimore recently published a systematic review of available literature investigating the nonoperative management of pseudoaneurysms and found only a 4% late intervention rate and 2% adjusted mortality rate. Although promising, the results of these studies are limited by the retrospective methodology used, small sample sizes and short-term follow-up, and more studies are needed before a nonoperative treatment strategy can be recommended widely. When applied, these patients should be closely followed with routine surveillance CT angiography of the chest; however, no consensus regarding the interval between imaging exist.

Once the need for repair has been determined, the timing of intervention is the next decision to be made. Owing to the typically high-energy blunt mechanisms that cause these injuries, a significant proportion of these patients have severe, life-threatening, multisystem injuries that increase their risk of perioperative morbidity and mortality. Early proponents of delayed repair suggested that, if other immediately life-threatening injures and their subsequent physiology could be ameliorated before intervention, outcomes of repair of BTAI may be improved. Several studies over the last 20 years have evaluated this concept.[19,22] In the multicenter AAST study, a significantly increased mortality was observed in patients undergoing early repair (16% vs 5.8%; odds ratio, 7.78),

Table 1 Society for Vascular Surgery grading system for BTAI	
Grade of BTAI	**Description**
I	Injuries confined to the intima.
II	Intramural hematomas or larger intimal flaps are present.
III	Presence of a pseudoaneurysm in which only the adventitia remains intact.
IV	Complete transection or rupture

Abbreviation: BTAI, blunt thoracic aortic injury.

despite both the early and the delayed procedure groups being comparable in terms of patient demographics, injury profiles, and method of repair. This mortality difference in patients undergoing early repair was also noted in a subgroup analysis of patients with major extrathoracic injuries (21% vs 3%), and trended this direction in those without major extrathoracic injuries, although it was not statistically significant. Furthermore, patients with major extrathoracic injuries also had lower rates of procedural complications, such as paraplegia and renal failure, when undergoing delayed repair. The data did show increased intensive care unit and hospital durations of stay; however, the authors concluded that, despite this difference, delayed repair was supported in all patients.[23] Currently, the Eastern Association for the Surgery of Trauma management guidelines published in 2015 suggest delayed repair, with the caveat that effective blood pressure control must be maintained.[6]

One of the more frequent concomitant injuries of concern with the management of BTAI is traumatic brain injury. Theoretic concerns while managing these injuries simultaneously include blood pressure parameters adversely affecting cerebral perfusion pressures and procedural anticoagulation that would worsen brain injury outcomes. Recently, a retrospective review by Rabin and colleagues[24] evaluated the effect of early versus delayed repair on progression on brain injury. They reported that 34% of patients undergoing early repair were noted to have neurologic deterioration after intervention, compared with 0% of those in the delayed repair group. The authors proposed that delayed repair with anticoagulation could be undertaken in 48 to 72 hours after injury once the traumatic brain injury was radiographically stable.

Open repair via thoracotomy occasionally requiring cardiopulmonary bypass was once the standard of care for BTAI (**Fig. 9**). However, it carried with it high rates of perioperative mortality, paraplegia, and blood loss.[14] In the early 1990s, the use of endovascular stent grafts emerged for the treatment of abdominal and thoracic aortic disease, and as early reports of improved outcomes emerged, these devices began being used for the treatment of aortic injury. The first direct comparison between open and endovascular repair was published by Ott and colleagues[25] in 2004, and although they presented a small sample size, their results trended toward improved outcomes in the endovascular group. Several years later, Demetriades and colleagues[8] published the first multicenter prospective study comparing open versus endovascular repair. This AAST-sponsored study included data from 18 centers and included 193

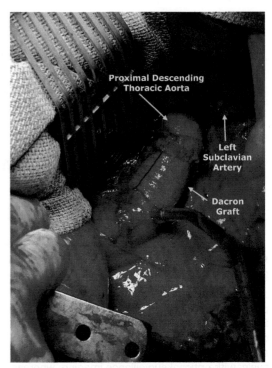

Fig. 9. Open descending thoracic aorta repair with interposition Dacron graft through a left posterolateral thoracotomy.

patients, 68 of whom were treated with open repair and 125 with endovascular stenting. Mortality in the endovascular repair group was significantly lower at 7.2% compared with 23.5% in the open repair group. The data also found overall lower rates of any systemic complications and a trend toward decreased procedure-related paraplegia for the endovascular technique. This study showed that, although once only recommended for high-risk patients, endovascular repair was progressively becoming the treatment of choice for all patient populations. Despite the improved outcomes, the authors did raise concern over high rates of device-related complications (20%), and cautioned about the lack of long-term data surrounding endografts, especially in young patients.

Subsequent studies have also supported these findings of improved outcomes associated with the endovascular repair of BTAI. In a single institution study, Azizzadeh and colleagues[26] demonstrated a 3-fold increase in complications or death for patients undergoing an open BTAI repair compared with their counterparts treated with an endovascular technique. In a follow-up AAST sponsored study, Dubose and colleagues[11] expanded on the previous 2008 study. Again, they noted that endovascular repair was protective of mortality, but also noted decreased device-related complications compared with the previous AAST study. The authors attributed this change to improvement of Food and Drug Administration–approved devices for this procedure. Based on the available evidence, treatment guidelines set forth by both the SVS and Eastern Association for the Surgery of Trauma recommend endovascular repair as treatment of choice over the open method.

At our institution, all patients admitted with a BTAI are primarily considered candidates for endovascular repair. The patients are admitted to the intensive care unit and strict blood pressure control is instituted. The initial chest CT scan is analyzed using commercially available DICOM imaging management software. Aortic diameters are recorded and 3-dimensional reconstruction and centerline measurements are performed allowing selection of the device to be used and planning of deployment location. After life-threatening associated injuries have been addressed, the patients undergo endovascular repair using percutaneous access. After femoral access is obtained and predeployment of suture-mediated closure devices are completed, a diagnostic angiogram is performed (**Figs. 10** and **11**). Intravascular ultrasound (IVUS) imaging is used routinely as an adjunct to assess the proximal and distal aortic diameters (**Figs. 12** and **13**), and to confirm the exact

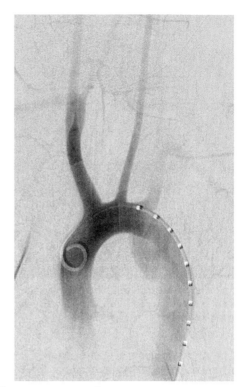

Fig. 11. Angiogram demonstrating proximal descending aorta pseudoaneurysm.

position of the arch branches (**Fig. 14**) and the location of the pseudoaneurysm (**Fig. 15**). The thoracic aortic endograft is then deployed and completion angiogram performed to confirm complete exclusion of the pseudoaneurysm (**Fig. 16**). Lumbar drain placement is reserved for patients

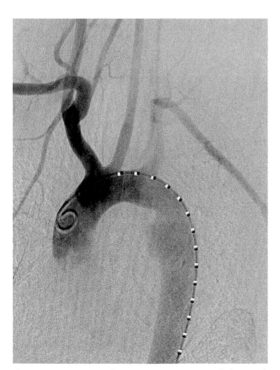

Fig. 10. Angiogram demonstrating proximal descending aorta pseudoaneurysm.

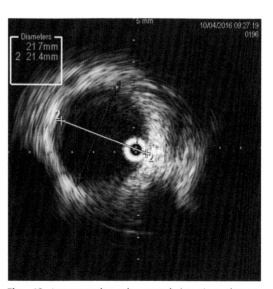

Fig. 12. Intravascular ultrasound imaging demonstrating procedural sizing of proximal aortic landing zone diameter.

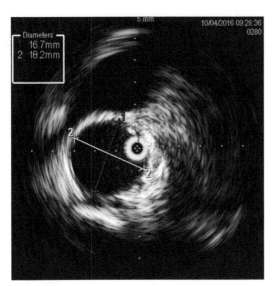

Fig. 13. Intravascular ultrasound imaging demonstrating procedural sizing of distal aortic landing zone diameter.

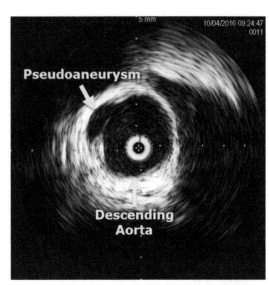

Fig. 15. Intravascular ultrasound imaging demonstrating an aortic pseudoaneurysm.

who develop symptoms of spinal ischemia, which is a rare occurrence. Postprocedural follow-up, including CT angiogram of the chest is important (**Fig. 17**); however, no consensus exist for the frequency at which imaging should be performed.

Although IVUS imaging is not universally adopted in endovascular aortic repair, it has a role as an adjunctive tool that can be used both for diagnostic purposes if CT imaging is not definitive or not safe in patients with renal insufficiency, or intraoperatively to aid with aortic sizing for

appropriate graft selection and ensure adequate landing zone distance for proximal seal. Two recent studies evaluating the benefit of IVUS imaging showed that, when compared with initial CT

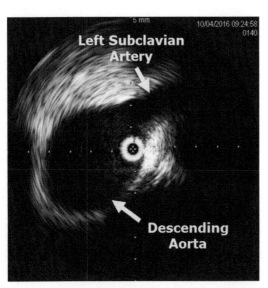

Fig. 14. Intravascular ultrasound imaging demonstrating the exact location of the aortic arch branch (left subclavian artery).

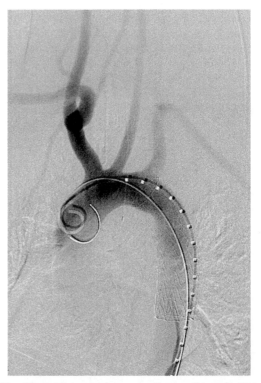

Fig. 16. Angiogram demonstrating aortic endostent graft deployed, with complete exclusion of the pseudoaneurysm.

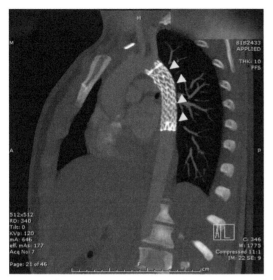

Fig. 17. Chest computed tomography scan, sagittal view, demonstrating a well-positioned proximal descending thoracic endostent graft (*arrowheads*), with complete exclusion of the pseudoaneurysm.

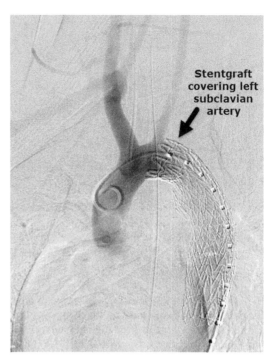

Fig. 18. Angiogram demonstrating aortic endostent graft deployed, requiring coverage of the ostium of the left subclavian artery for adequate proximal seal and complete exclusion of the pseudoaneurysm.

scan, aortic diameter on IVUS imaging was larger.[27,28] The authors attributed these findings to changes in hemodynamic status and resuscitation and noted that graft size determined based on CT scan images was changed in approximately one-half of the patients based on IVUS measurements. This procedure can theoretically lead to more accurate device sizing with consequent better seal and reduced rate of endoleaks, and a lower risk of graft migration or collapse.

Owing to the usual location of the BTAI just distal to the left subclavian artery (LSA), coverage of the LSA ostium may be necessary to achieve the proximal seal (**Fig. 18**). The potential risks associated with LSA coverage acutely include stroke, spinal ischemia, and cardiac ischemia in patients who have undergone coronary bypass grafting using the left internal mammary artery as a conduit, and at a later phase subclavian steal syndrome and left arm pain from arterial insufficiency. Despite these considerations, the published literature has shown that coverage of the LSA is commonly done and well-tolerated, without significantly increased risk of ischemic symptom or need for revascularization.[11,29,30] Currently, the SVS guidelines suggest against routine revascularization, instead proposing a selective approach based on the status of vertebral anatomy dominance and the circle of Willis.[14] Options in the event that revascularization is needed include carotid–subclavian bypass (**Fig. 19**) or subclavian–carotid transposition (**Fig. 20**).

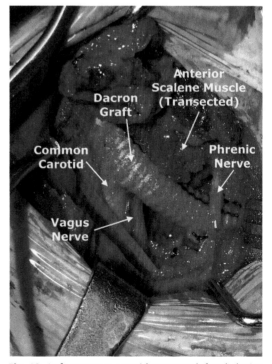

Fig. 19. Left common carotid artery to left subclavian artery bypass through a left supraclavicular access.

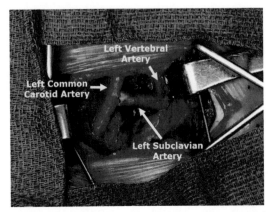

Fig. 20. Left subclavian artery to left common carotid artery transposition through a left supraclavicular access.

SUMMARY

BTAI remains a major cause of prehospital deaths. For patients who reach the hospital alive, the diagnosis and management of this injury have undergone dramatic changes over the last 50 years. CT scanning is the imaging modality of choice for injury diagnosis and repair planning. The implementation of medical management with antihypertensives dramatically decreased the risk of rupture, allowing for delayed repair while abnormal physiology and more immediately life-threatening injuries can be addressed. With the advent of endovascular techniques and ongoing progress in endograft technology, the risks associated with repair of this injury have reduced significantly, and this treatment modality has become the standard of care. Owing to a lack of long-term follow-up, however, the incidence of late complications associated with the devices currently available is not known.

REFERENCES

1. Demetriades D, Talving P, Inaba K. Blunt thoracic aortic injury. In: Rich's vascular trauma. Elsevier; 2016. p. 100–12.
2. Parmley LF, Mattingly TW, Manion WC, et al. Nonpenetrating traumatic injury of the aorta. Circulation 1958;17(6):1086–101.
3. Passaro E, Pace WG. Traumatic rupture of the aorta. Surgery 1959;46:787–91.
4. Kato N, Dake MD, Miller DC, et al. Traumatic thoracic aortic aneurysm: treatment with endovascular stent-grafts. Radiology 1997;205(3):657–62.
5. Demetriades D, Velmahos GC, Scalea TM, et al. Diagnosis and treatment of blunt thoracic aortic injuries: changing perspectives. J Trauma Acute Care Surg 2008;64(6):1415–8 [discussion: 1418–9].
6. Fox N, Schwartz D, Salazar JH, et al. Evaluation and management of blunt traumatic aortic injury. J Trauma Acute Care Surg 2015;78(1):136–46.
7. Arthurs ZM, Starnes BW, Sohn VY, et al. Functional and survival outcomes in traumatic blunt thoracic aortic injuries: an analysis of the National Trauma Databank. J Vasc Surg 2009;49(4):988–94.
8. Demetriades D, Velmahos GC, Scalea TM, et al. Operative repair or endovascular stent graft in blunt traumatic thoracic aortic injuries: results of an American Association for the Surgery of Trauma Multicenter Study. J Trauma Acute Care Surg 2008; 64(3):561–70 [discussion: 570–1].
9. Teixeira PGR, Inaba K, Barmparas G, et al. Blunt thoracic aortic injuries: an autopsy study. J Trauma Acute Care Surg 2011;70(1):197–202.
10. Burkhart HM, Gomez GA, Jacobson LE, et al. Fatal blunt aortic injuries: a review of 242 autopsy cases. J Trauma 2001;50(1):113–5.
11. Dubose JJ, Leake SS, Brenner M, et al. Contemporary management and outcomes of blunt thoracic aortic injury: a multicenter retrospective study. J Trauma Acute Care Surg 2015;78(2):360–9.
12. Ekeh AP, Peterson W, Woods RJ, et al. Is chest X-Ray an adequate screening tool for the diagnosis of blunt thoracic aortic injury? J Trauma Acute Care Surg 2008;65(5):1088–92.
13. Gutierrez A, Inaba K, Siboni S, et al. The utility of chest X-ray as a screening tool for blunt thoracic aortic injury. Injury 2016;47(1):32–6.
14. Lee WAW, Matsumura JSJ, Mitchell RSR, et al. Endovascular repair of traumatic thoracic aortic injury: clinical practice guidelines of the Society for Vascular Surgery. J Vasc Surg 2011;53(1):187–92.
15. Heneghan RE, Aarabi S, Quiroga E, et al. Call for a new classification system and treatment strategy in blunt aortic injury. J Vasc Surg 2016;64(1):171–6.
16. Fabian TC, Davis KA, Gavant ML, et al. Prospective study of blunt aortic injury. Ann Surg 1998;227(5): 666–77.
17. Akins CW, Buckley MJ, Daggett W, et al. Acute traumatic disruption of the thoracic aorta: a ten-year experience. Ann Thorac Surg 1981;31(4):305–9.
18. Warren RL, Akins CW, Conn AK, et al. Acute traumatic disruption of the thoracic aorta: emergency department management. Ann Emerg Med 1992; 21(4):391–6.
19. Maggisano R, Maggisano R, Nathens A, et al. Traumatic rupture of the thoracic aorta: should one always operate immediately? Ann Vasc Surg 1995;9(1):44–52.
20. Demetriades D. Blunt thoracic aortic injuries: crossing the Rubicon. J Am Coll Surg 2012;214(3):247–59.
21. Harris DG, Rabin J, Bhardwaj A, et al. Nonoperative management of traumatic aortic pseudoaneurysms. Ann Vasc Surg 2016;35:75–81.
22. Hemmila MR, Arbabi S, Rowe SA, et al. Delayed repair for blunt thoracic aortic injury: is it really

equivalent to early repair? J Trauma Acute Care Surg 2004;56(1):13–23.

23. Demetriades D, Velmahos GC, Scalea TM, et al. Blunt traumatic thoracic aortic injuries: early or delayed repair–results of an American Association for the Surgery of Trauma prospective study. J Trauma Acute Care Surg 2009;66(4):967–73.

24. Rabin J, Harris DG, Crews GA, et al. Early aortic repair worsens concurrent traumatic brain injury. Ann Thorac Surg 2014;98(1):46–52.

25. Ott MC, Stewart TC, Lawlor DK, et al. Management of blunt thoracic aortic injuries: endovascular stents versus open repair. J Trauma 2004;56(3):565–70.

26. Azizzadeh A, Charlton-Ouw KM, Chen Z, et al. An outcome analysis of endovascular versus open repair of blunt traumatic aortic injuries. J Vasc Surg 2013;57(1):108–15.

27. Shi Y, Tsai PI, Wall MJ Jr, et al. Intravascular ultrasound enhanced aortic sizing for endovascular treatment of blunt aortic injury. J Trauma Acute Care Surg 2015;79(5):817–21.

28. Wallace GA, Starnes BW, Hatsukami TS, et al. Intravascular ultrasound is a critical tool for accurate endograft sizing in the management of blunt thoracic aortic injury. J Vasc Surg 2015;61(3):630–5.

29. Azizzadeh A, Ray HM, Dubose JJ, et al. Outcomes of endovascular repair for patients with blunt traumatic aortic injury. J Trauma Acute Care Surg 2014;76(2):510–6.

30. McBride CL, Dubose JJ, Miller CC, et al. Intentional left subclavian artery coverage during thoracic endovascular aortic repair for traumatic aortic injury. J Vasc Surg 2015;61(1):73–9.

Neuroprotection Strategies in Aortic Surgery

Edward J. Bergeron, MD[a], Matthew S. Mosca, CCP[b],
Muhammad Aftab, MD[a], George Justison, CCP[c],
Thomas Brett Reece, MD[a],*

KEYWORDS

- Neuroprotection • Neurologic monitoring • Brain oximetry • Near-infrared spectroscopy
- Deep hypothermic circulatory arrest • Circulatory arrest • Antegrade cerebral perfusion
- Retrograde cerebral perfusion

KEY POINTS

- Common modalities of neuromonitoring used in aortic arch surgery are electroencephalography (EEG), peripheral somatosensory-evoked potentials (SEPs), and cerebral oximetry by near-infrared spectroscopy (NIRS).
- Selective antegrade cerebral perfusion (sACP) typically involves cannulation of the right innominate or axillary artery with simultaneous clamping of the more proximal innominate artery. The resulting cerebral blood flow (CBF) is via the right carotid artery, whereas the remainder of the body undergoes circulatory arrest. An intact circle of Willis is mandated for the unilaterally antegrade cannulated innominate or axillary artery to provide contralateral cerebral hemisphere flow.
- Adjunctive cerebral perfusion results in adequate brain protection at more moderate hypothermic temperatures resulting in decreased hypothermia-related coagulopathy, decreased cardiopulmonary bypass (CPB) times, decreased renal dysfunction, and decreased hypothermia-related neuronal injury.
- Two acid-base management strategies exist, alpha stat and pH stat. Each offers distinct advantages and is implemented during particular stages of hypothermic CPB.
- The benefits associated with inducing lower body circulatory arrest at more moderate degrees of hypothermia will likely continue the current trend of increasing moderate hypothermic circulatory arrest (MHCA) with sACP adoption.

INTRODUCTION

Surgical therapy for aortic arch dissections and aneurysms involves partial or complete replacement of the aortic arch. Intervention requires anatomic-specific consideration for the aorta and its affected organ systems, specifically, the potential for neurologic risks or perioperative effects. Neurologic protection during aortic arch surgery is challenging due to the 3 branches from the aortic arch giving rise to the vessels completely

Disclosures: The authors have no disclosures.
[a] Thoracic Aortic Surgery Program, Division of Cardiothoracic Surgery, Department of Surgery, University of Colorado Anschutz Medical Campus, 12631 East 17th Avenue, C-310, Aurora, CO 80045, USA; [b] Perfusion Services, University of Colorado Hospital, 12605 East 16th Avenue, Mail Stop B200, Aurora, CO 80045, USA; [c] Perfusion Services, Perioperative Services, University of Colorado Hospital, 12605 East 16th Avenue, Mail Stop B200, Aurora, CO 80045, USA
* Corresponding author.
E-mail address: Brett.Reece@ucdenver.edu

responsible for brain perfusion. Nervous tissue is particularly at risk during aortic procedures due to its high metabolic demand and dependence on aerobic metabolism. The potential for devastating, and potentially irreversible, neurologic-related morbidity resulting from ischemic injury to the brain and spinal cord mandates that neuroprotection is the principal concern during circulatory management in aortic surgery. The entire spectrum of neurologic injury, from transient paresis to stroke or paraplegia, is possible in aortic surgery. Hemiarch and total aortic arch replacements necessitate an open distal anastomosis and circulatory arrest. This requirement results in either ischemic visceral beds, or at least a decreased level of perfusion perioperatively. As a result, strategies have been developed to minimize neurologic injury from hypoperfusion and to lengthen circulatory arrest times while maintaining a margin of safety. These strategies include pharmacologic adjuncts, hypothermic circulatory arrest (HCA), antegrade cerebral perfusion (ACP), and retrograde cerebral perfusion (RCP). Monitoring is a key component of surgery, both intraoperatively and postoperatively, for optimal outcomes.

This review discusses the methods of neuroprotection during aortic arch procedures. These involve pharmacology, cooling, neuromonitoring, and circulatory and cannulation management strategies, allowing for actively manipulating CBF to circulatory arrest, rewarming, and acid-base management.

PROCEDURAL OF RISKS

Diseases of the ascending and aortic arch include acute aortic dissection to chronic aneurysmal disease. Aortic arch surgery, when performed for these diseases, puts patients at multiple risks. Although this review focuses on neurologic risks (**Table 1**), the risks of myocardial infarction, perioperative respiratory insufficiency, and renal dysfunction are also common. The disease process combined with the surgical repair of aortic arch diseases may involve any component of the circulation, resulting in potential visceral bed malperfusion to the heart, brain, spinal cord, kidneys, gastrointestinal tract, and extremities. Because current trends are for aortic repairs performed at more moderate temperatures that may mitigate theoretic systemic complications of deeper hypothermia (ie, renal dysfunction and bleeding complications), adjuncts must be incorporated to maintain or decrease current neurologic risk profiles. Prolonged CPB time is a risk factor for the development of bilateral watershed strokes, perhaps the result of increased

---

Table 1
Independent predictors of neurologic dysfunction specific to arch and ascending aorta surgery.

Stroke	Temporary Neurologic Dysfunction
Age (>60 y old)	Age
Female	Prior stroke/TIA
History of cerebrovascular disease	History of central neurologic event
New preoperative neurologic symptoms	Estimated GFR <90 mL/min
Hypertension	Emergency operation status
Diabetes	Acute type A dissection
Chronic obstructive pulmonary disease	Proximal aortic surgery
Previous aortic surgery distal to the left subclavian artery	Duration of cardiac arrest
Emergency operation status	Total cerebral protection time
Acute type A dissection	Concomitant cardiac procedures (ie, coronary artery bypass grafting)
Operation intended for the arch (including total arch replacement)	Red blood cell transfusion
Descending aortic aneurysm containing clot/atheroma	
General presence of clot/atheroma in aorta	
CPB time	
Duration of cardiac arrest	
Total cerebral protection time	
History of cerebral infarction or transient ischemic attack	
Concomitant cardiac procedures (ie, mitral valve replacement)	

Abbreviations: GFR, glomerular filtration rate; TIA, transient ischemic attack.

opportunity for hypoperfusion during longer CPB. The need for cooling also places the patient at risk for bleeding complications, primarily from platelet dysfunction. In cases of acute aortic dissection, the emergent nature of the operation also increases the risk profile for the patient.

The need for concomitant cardiac procedures (ie, valve replacement or repair and coronary artery bypass grafting) also increases risk for the patient.

PHARMACOLOGY

With aortic arch reconstruction and the associated circulatory arrest, there are several pharmaco-therapies that may diminish neurologic injury. Although no randomized prospective trials exist that prove the following drugs are beneficial, there is some animal evidence suggesting benefit. **Table 2** summarizes the drugs that have been suggested for use in aortic arch surgeries. More specifically, the drugs discussed are commonly used as part of the authors' institutional protocol.

Steroids

Steroids given before CPB are thought to decrease brain damage by decreasing the proin-flammatory response. Furthermore, there is some evidence that some steroids can act as antioxi-dants for the ischemic tissues. The associated hy-perglycemia, however, must be monitored and treated aggressively.[1]

Lidocaine

Lidocaine is thought to improve neurocognitive outcomes by decreasing the cerebral metabolic rate of oxygen.

Magnesium

Magnesium may be protective by decreasing the voltage-sensitive and N-methyl-D-aspartate (NMDA)-activated calcium channels. Reduction in vasospasm may also be beneficial.[2]

Dexmedetomidine

Dexmedetomidine inhibits ischemia-induced norepinephrine release.

At the authors' institution, a majority of circula-tory arrest cases receive 500 mg of methylprednis-olone after induction of anesthesia, followed by 100 mg of lidocaine and 2 g of magnesium during the cooling phase of CPB when 28°C is reached. Dexmedetomidine is commonly used in the imme-diate postoperative period.[3]

Table 2
Summary of drugs experimentally suggested for neuroprotection in aortic reconstructions. The evidence for pharmacologically neuroprotective drugs is weak

Human Guidelines	Human Studies	Animal Studies
Glucocorticoids, high-dose (intravenous)	Naloxone (intravenous)	Aprotinin
Mannitol	Papaverine (intrathecal)	Opioids (morphine)
	Lidocaine	Methylprednisone (intrathecal)
	Magnesium sulfate	Defurozamine (DFOA, Desferal)
	Barbiturates (thiopental)	Superoxide dismutase
		Minocycline
		Erythropoietin
		Testosterone
		Dexmedetomidine
		Propofol
		α-Blockers
		Nimodipine
		Nicardipine
		Phenytoin
		Midazolam
		Propofol
		Fentanyl
		Isoflurane
		Diazoxide
		Insulin
		Cyclosporin A
		Fructose 1,6-bisphosphonate
		GM1-ganglioside

NEUROMONITORING/NEUROPHYSIOLOGIC INTRAOPERATIVE MONITORING

The common modalities of neuromonitoring used during surgery of the aortic arch are EEG, peripheral SEPs, and cerebral oximetry by NIRS. These technologies are collectively termed, *neurophysiologic intraoperative monitoring* (*NIOM*). NIOM is often used during aortic arch procedures to provide simultaneous, real-time assessments of cerebral status and direct intraoperative decisions on the circulatory management and neuroprotective adjustment strategies during these procedures.[4]

Electroencephalography

EEG is the primary NIOM modality used during surgery of the aortic arch. Baseline EEG readings should be obtained after anesthetic induction but before the initiation of CPB cooling. Electrocerebral activity is heavily influenced by anesthesia. This reference EEG is important for the identification of any baseline asymmetry or abnormality that may not have had a preoperative clinical correlation on physical examination or in situations where obtaining a baseline neurologic examination was limited (ie, acute type A dissections).

Next, continuous EEG monitoring is initiated with onset of CPB. The EEG likely exhibits higher amplitude prior to cooling, but once cooling is initiated the EEG amplitude diminishes. Correct monitoring includes sensitivity adjustment for the detection of this cooling-related lower-amplitude waveform. The EEG is then continuously monitored throughout the process of cooling to provide intraoperative real-time assessment of the electrocerebral activity. This electrocerebral activity of the brain serves as a surrogate for hypothermia-mediated metabolic suppression of the brain. Once cooling is initiated, anesthetics are typically discontinued in efforts not to confound the impact that the anesthetic agents have on EEG interpretation with hypothermia. The institutional anesthesia protocol is an important consideration with EEG monitoring when used in conjunction with cooling for aortic arch procedures.

EEG electrocerebral activity progresses through a series of predictable waveforms phases during cooling[5] and rewarming[6] for HCA. To summarize, a burst suppression pattern becomes present between 15.7°C and 33.0°C (mean 24.4°C) and progression to complete electrocerebral inactivity (ECI) is typically accomplished from 12.5°C and 27.2°C (mean 17.8°C). During patient rewarming, a reversed progression from ECI back to the normal amplitude continuous activity occurs. Although the phases of the waveforms are predictable during rewarming, the particular temperature points at which these EEG patterns change differ in comparison to the process of cooling. The temperature points at which the predictable pattern of electrocerebral activity progresses during cooling and rewarming varies widely.

Distinct from cooling-related changes in electrocerebral activity, the cooling rates of the body are also not uniform and depend on several patient and procedural factors.[7] Surface and core temperature measurements are recognized as poor surrogates for brain temperature.[8] Subsequently, it is not possible to predict the extent or duration of the cooling required for specific changes in electrocerebral activity for any particular patient. Thus, the importance of NIOM during aortic arch surgery is necessitated for the real-time acquisition of electrocerebral activity. The related brain metabolism can only be known by direct monitoring.

The optimal temperature and degree of hypothermia prior to initiation of circulatory arrest are unknown and remain topics of debate among aortic surgeons. The most common traditional strategy for circulatory management was cooling the patient to the point of ECI just prior to circulatory arrest. Cooling to ECI was thought to ensure optimal neuroprotection from the circulatory arrest–related ischemic insult because ECI correlates with the minimal cerebral metabolic demand threshold.[9]

Somatosensory-evoked potentials

Median nerve SEPs can be monitored during surgery of the aortic arch with HCA. The body of literature examining SEPs in comparison to EEG is small.[4] Cortical, subcortical, and peripheral responses can be monitored intraoperatively to provide information on brain activity through the process of cooling. The cortical responses are the first to be lost, followed by the subcortical responses and finally the peripheral responses. These responses may be used to demonstrate cerebral metabolic suppression before the initiation of circulatory arrest and may help to guide MHCP–ACP therapy.

Near-infrared spectroscopy

NIRS cerebral oximetry is another adjunctive NIOM technique used in surgery of the aortic arch.[10] This technology was developed in the 1970s and allows for the determination of regional cerebral oxygen saturation ($rScO_2$) by measuring the different absorptive properties of saturated and unsaturated hemoglobin in the near-infrared spectrum.[11]

The vast majority of the literature relating to NIRS for NIOM comes from experimental animal models and pediatric cardiac surgery, where the use of NIRS for NIOM during CPB, especially during circulatory arrest, has become common. There is significantly less literature relating to NIRS in adult cardiac surgery.[12] NIRS is a noninvasive technique with simple interpretation that is easily applied to the surgical patient. NIRS is a crucial NIOM adjunct, allowing the surgical team, in a data-guided method to navigate through the complex circulatory management required for aortic arch surgery. As a result, NIRS is increasingly used,[13] and early studies have supported NIRS as a potentially viable NIOM modality during aortic arch reconstructions in adults.[14,15]

Studies have demonstrated that $rScO_2$ remains stable on the initiation of cooling and may actually increase from basal levels. After the initiation of circulatory arrest, the tissue oxygenation levels steadily decline until circulation is restored.[16] The extent of tissue hypoxia, as determined by NIRS, correlates with the severity of neurologic tissue damage.[17] Additionally, NIRS serves a role in detecting potential situations of contralateral regional brain ischemia during unilateral selective ACP. Although the NIRS hints are not absolute for regional brain ischemia, they allow for immediate, intraoperative actionable perfusion strategies, such as implementation of bilateral ACP to restore contralateral tissue oxygenation.[15,18]

Concerns regarding the utility of NIRS remain, particularly in adult patients. The larger cerebral volume and mass of interfering tissue may interfere with the NIRS's reliability of deeper brain tissue oxygenation determinations. Historically, NIRS determined $rScO_2$ has poor correlation with jugular venous bulb saturation, a largely historical surrogate for cerebral oxygenation during aortic arch surgery.[19] Despite these NIRS concerns, currently no data suggest a threshold saturation level or duration time of NIRS-determined brain hypoxia tolerated without detrimental neurocognitive effects. Subsequently, NIRS-directed circulatory management decisions based on $rScO_2$ remain nebulous. The authors' adult aortic arch surgery institutional experience, with which EEG, SEP, and NIRS are all used concurrently, is that NIRS is less sensitive and less specific than EEG in the detection of real-time brain ischemia but still a useful adjunct to guide operations and help patient welfare.

DEEP HYPOTHERMIC CIRCULATORY ARREST

Several aortic arch surgical series have demonstrated good perioperative outcomes with low rates of neurologic morbidity and mortality, using a circulatory management strategy cooling the patient to a temperature where ECI is accomplished prior to the induction of circulatory arrest.[20–25] This method is referred to as deep HCA (DHCA). With DHCA, low degrees of hypothermia are required to reach ECI. This strategy requires longer periods of cooling and more severe hypothermia in comparison to alternative circulatory management strategies.

MODERATE HYPOTHERMIC CIRCULATORY PERFUSION WITH SELECTIVE ANTEGRADE CEREBRAL PERFUSION/MODERATE HYPOTHERMIC CIRCULATORY PERFUSION WITH RETROGRADE CEREBRAL PERFUSION

Although the field of aortic arch surgery was founded with a DHCA circulatory management strategy, an increasing number of aortic surgery centers are shifting from DHCA in favor of initiating circulatory arrest at more moderate degrees of hypothermia, before ECI is achieved.[26–28] Several factors are responsible for the shift away from DHCA when patient criteria allow. The increasing role and experience with ACP and RCP during lower body circulatory arrest are likely the most noteworthy factors.[29,30] With ACP, the brain is continuously perfused resulting in adequate brain protection at more moderate hypothermic temperatures than with the DHCA temperatures required for ECI. Initiating systemic circulatory arrest at more moderate temperatures results in decreased hypothermia-related coagulopathy, decreased CPB times, decreased renal dysfunction, and decreased hypothermia-related neuronal injury.[31,32] This circulatory management strategy is known as MHCA–sACP. Its neurologic outcomes are comparable to the more traditional DHCA approach.[26–28,33] The benefits associated with inducing lower body circulatory arrest at more moderate degrees of hypothermia will likely continue the current trend of increasing MHCA–sACP adoption.

When an MHCA–ACP circulatory management strategy is used, the temperature at which circulatory arrest is initiated is arbitrarily selected, typically based on aortic surgery centers' experiences and associated biases (there is great variability in the current literature regarding the temperatures referred to as moderate hypothermia, in addition to the location of the temperature measurement).[34] A majority of patients continue to demonstrate electrocerebral activity at these moderate temperatures, and the electrophysiologic behavior of the brain near the time of circulatory arrest and initiation of ACP remains in the discovery phase. Unlike DHCA, where NIOM has been used to specifically inform the timing of circulatory arrest initiation, the role of NIOM with MHCA–ACP is not clearly defined. Data suggest, however, that the use of EEG monitoring in MHCA may help with intraoperative identification of electrocerebral asymmetry or abrupt loss of electrocerebral activity after circulatory arrest that is not restored by the establishment of ACP. In these circumstances, EEG data allow for real-time intraoperative adjustment of neuroprotective strategies, including reinitiation of circulatory support with additional cooling or transition to bilateral ACP to address asymmetric EEG changes.[35]

From a purely published, evidence-based perspective, the utility of NIOM during the surgery of the ascending aorta and aortic arch is unproved. To date, there are no comparative studies examining the effect of EEG on outcomes of aortic arch surgery, regardless of circulatory management strategy. Early evidence suggesting, however, that EEG during MHCA–ACP may be useful in identifying changes in electrocerebral activity concerning for ischemia leading to potential corrective intraoperative adjustments will continue to value the role of EEG toward optimizing patient outcomes, as the field continues to trend away from the traditional DHCA circulatory management strategy.[34]

PERFUSION/CEREBRAL BLOOD FLOW MANAGEMENT

CPB can significantly impair CBF autoregulation. CBF, then, depends on mean arterial pressure (MAP). Thus, a low MAP can cause hypoperfusion and subsequent cerebral ischemia. A high MAP can cause increased intracerebral pressure and resulting cerebral edema. Impairment of cerebral autoregulation has been reported in up to 20% of CPB cases.[36] This is particularly evident during rewarming.

HCA and its effects on CBF autoregulation was specifically investigated for patients undergoing aortic reconstruction. HCA did not seem to adversely affect CBF autoregulation compared with standard cooling methods. HCA and related perfusion techniques may be protective against impaired autoregulation during rewarming compared with the non-HCA group.[37]

CANNULATION

As with the other components of aortic arch surgery, cannulation has evolved to improve patient outcomes, including the prevention of neurologic sequelae. The ascending aorta has traditionally been the site for CPB cannulation.[38] This site can be complicated, however, by dissection, aneurysms, and thrombotic disease, all of which can result in embolism or malperfusion. Concern

for posterior cerebral circulation compromise with primary innominate artery and carotid artery cannulation has also been investigated.[39] Although axillary artery cannulation is recommended by some current guidelines, the predominating factor is surgeon preference after consideration for underlying pathology and atheroma or clot burden by epiaortic or transesophageal echocardiogram. The basis for the recommendation of axillary or subclavian artery cannulation allows for the potential benefits of sACP and avoiding potential degradation of an atherosclerotic lined aortic endothelium.[40] This recommendation is evidence based, from only observational studies.[41] The authors typically use a cannulation technique with an interposed graft sewn directly to the vessel.

The femoral artery, an alternative site, has traditionally been favored when rapid CPB commencement and prompt cooling are needed in emergent cases. Femoral cannulation has been studied and compared with central cannulation (ascending aorta, innominate artery, and right axillary artery) with results showing no difference in neurologic outcomes.[39]

ANTEGRADE CEREBRAL PERFUSION

The concept of antegrade cerebral perfusion was first introduced in the subspecialty of aortic surgery in 1957.[42] It has since been iterated and commonly includes hypothermia with ongoing partial directional CBF. Typical minimal antegrade cerebral flowrates of 6 mL/kg/min to 10 mL/kg/min and pressures of 40 mm Hg to 60 mm Hg are used. sACP most typically involves cannulation of the right innominate or axillary artery with simultaneous clamping of the more proximal innominate artery. The resulting CBF is via the right carotid artery, whereas the remainder of the body undergoes circulatory arrest.[43–45] An intact circle of Willis is mandated for the unilaterally antegrade cannulated innominate or axillary artery to provide contralateral cerebral hemisphere flow. Subsequently, patients with ipsilateral carotid artery stenosis or an incomplete circle of Willis (described in up to 20% of patients[46]) are contraindicated for this technique. NIRS monitoring is used during unilateral ACP as a surrogate of cerebral perfusion, and to detect cannula malposition that may occur throughout the procedure.[47] Disadvantages of ACP include vessel stenosis secondary to (de)cannulation, vessel wall damage from excessive perfusion pressure, risk of air and/or plaque embolization, and cerebral edema from hyperperfusion. Despite multiple studies, there has been no significant difference in outcomes between unilateral ACP and bilateral ACP with regard to cerebral morbidity or overall mortality.[33]

RETROGRADE CEREBRAL PERFUSION

RCP is used at some centers to prevent the brain from rewarming during circulatory arrest periods and, in theory, to wash out any particulate or gaseous emboli. RCP involves cannulating the superior vena cava and perfusing retrograde with oxygenated blood. RCP flow is instituted with the goal to raise the central venous pressure to 25 mm Hg with 300 mL/min to 500 mL/min of cerebral flow. Like sACP, RCP results in a separate cerebral perfusion circuit, while simultaneously the rest of the lower body remains in HCA.

Additionally, the original theory of RCP was that it could extend the safe period of circulatory arrest by providing metabolic support and catabolite removal for the brain. This theory of metabolic benefit via brain capillary retrograde blood flow has been questioned in published animal studies.[48] Experimentally, significant shunting of venous flow among various venous systems, including between the internal and external jugular vein to the azygous vein and cerebral sinuses, occurs resulting in lacking cerebral perfusion. Furthermore, there are more than 20 such venovenous anastomoses in humans.[49] Thus, clinical studies portray benefit from RCP thought to result primarily from maintenance of brain hypothermia via continuous perfusion with cold blood, rather than from metabolic support. Any slow rise in temperature can likely be prevented safely, simply by thorough initial cooling and packing the head with ice. Finally, there are concerns that RCP may actually worsen neurologic outcomes by inducing cerebral edema. Two small clinical studies have shown that RCP did not provide significant metabolic assistance or improve neuropsychological outcomes.[50,51]

HYPOTHERMIC CIRCULATORY ARREST

Hypothermia reduces considerably the metabolic demands of tissues by reducing their enzymatic activity. Specifically in the brain, hypothermia also reduces the release of glutamate, an excitatory neurotransmitter. As a general rule, for every 1°C below 37°C there is a 6% to 7% decrease in metabolism.[52] During aortic surgery, HCA involves cooling the brain and body using the CPB circuit before circulatory arrest. This CPB cooling combined with packing a patient's head with ice reduces cerebral metabolic demand for an interval to complete the aortic arch repair.[53] Clinical studies have used varying definitions and classifications for graded hypothermia temperatures. The current

consensus statement among aortic surgeons defines hypothermia as mild (28.1°C–34°C), moderate (20.1°C–28°C [MHCA]), deep (14.1°C–20°C [DHCA]), and profound ($\leq$14°C)[34] (**Table 3**).

In a series of 616 aortic surgery patients using DHCA, Svensson and colleagues[22] found a stroke rate of 7%, with a mean DHCA time of 31 minutes (range, 7–120 min). DHCA times greater than 45 minutes and greater than 60 minutes were independent predictors of stroke and early mortality, respectively, with univariate analyses. Other studies have shown DHCA duration of 25 minutes is associated with increased risks of memory, fine motor, and transient neurologic deficits.[54,55] Electrocerebral silence is achieved in only 2% to 25% of patients cooled to 20°C and 78% to 86% at 14.1°C.[34] Thus, the authors regularly use the aid of pharmacology, specifically propofol, to help with electrocerebral silence with DHCA, even at temperatures more moderate than DHCA. For this incomplete role of temperature with electrocerebral silence, DHCA provides for a limited time frame to perform aortic arch procedures. It provides for well-tolerated circulatory arrest times of approximately 20 minutes to 30 minutes before prolonged postoperative impairment in memory and fine motor function occurs. If DHCA is to be used as the sole perfusion strategy (without sACP or RCP), then it only should be used when the anticipated circulatory arrest duration is less than 30 minutes.

Profound hypothermia ($\leq$14°C) is not routinely used for several intentions. Physiologically, between the cerebral temperatures of 10°C and 15°C, the cerebral metabolic rate minimally increases from 11% to 16%, for a total of 5%.[56] Additionally, there is significant increased risk of platelet dysfunction and coagulopathy as a major morbidity of profound hypothermia.[57] Decreased immune system response and subsequent increased risk of infection are also exacerbated with these colder temperatures[58] as are the longer CPB and overall operating room times it requires

Table 3	
Aortic arch hypothermia classification consensus temperatures	
Category	**Nasopharyngeal Temperature**
Mild hypothermia	34°C–28.1°C
Moderate hypothermia	28°C–20.1°C
Deep hypothermia	20°C–14.1°C
Profound hypothermia	$\leq$14°C

to cool and rewarm a patient to these more extreme temperatures. In summary, profound hypothermia does not confer clinically significant physiologic advantage versus the substantial clinical patient risks compared with DHCA.

TOPICAL HEAD COOLING/SURFACE COOLING

Despite the almost ubiquitous practice of topical head cooling, and more generally surface cooling, at aortic surgery centers around the world, there is limited published evidence of its efficacy in clinical application.[59] Those investigators in favor of the practice suggest that it prevents rebound rewarming during cardiac arrest and helps ensure uniform cerebral hypothermia in the minority of patients with nonimaged but imperfect cerebral circulations.[60] Antagonists of topical head and surface cooling suggest the theoretic risks of pressure injury, thermal injury, and retinal ischemia.[61] There are no human clinical outcome trials supporting these arguments.

ACID-BASE MANAGEMENT

Currently, there is no consensus on the optimal acid-base management strategy for adult cardiac surgery patients who are cooled to more than moderate hypothermia ($<28°C$) and undergo a period of HCA. Two acid-base managements strategies exist, alpha stat and pH stat, and each offers distinct advantages when implemented during certain stages of hypothermic CPB. The aim of alpha stat is to keep a nontemperature corrected pH of 7.4 and a Pco_2 of 40 mm Hg irrespective of a patient's actual body temperature. This technique conserves the ionization of the imidazole groups on intracellular proteins and maintains intracellular electrochemical neutrality,[62] buffering, and enzymatic function.[63] The aim of pH stat is to keep a temperature corrected (the patient's actual blood temperature) pH of 7.4 and a Pco_2 of 40 mm Hg. This practice compensates for the decreased blood Pco_2 induced by hypothermia and increased CO_2 solubility.

The authors' acid-base management protocol on CPB for cases cooling below 28°C with a period of circulatory arrest uses both alpha stat and pH stat to optimize cerebral protection. CPB is initiated with alpha stat management. During active cooling, a pH stat management is switched to by reducing the gas–to–blood flow ratio of the oxygenator to retain carbon dioxide. This pH stat technique is maintained during HCA and antegrade cerebral perfusion. Immediately on systemic reperfusion, an alpha stat management is switched to for the remainder of the rewarming

period. Aggressive oxygenator gas flow is used to quickly remove the retained carbon dioxide in the early reperfusion period.

The use of alpha stat on CPB initiation conserves imidazole-buffering capacity and may prevent intracellular derangements as the patient begins to cool. It also allows the perfusionist time to respond to any abnormal blood gas results prior to initiating pH stat. Alpha stat may be associated with higher cerebral oxygenation at mild hypothermia compared with pH stat.[64] Beyond the initial blood gas, if alpha stat is used during cooling to circulatory arrest, the nontemperature corrected blood gas yields a lower $Paco_2$ and the blood is alkaline relative to a temperature corrected (pH stat) blood gas. A lower $Paco_2$ may induce cerebral vasoconstriction and cause ischemia in poorly perfused regions of the brain. Blood alkalosis shifts the oxyhemoglobin curve to the left decreasing oxygen unloading at the tissues. This effect may be offset by higher amounts of oxygen dissolved in the plasma at hypothermia, but the net effect is not well studied.

Using pH stat during the cooling period permits a normal $Paco_2$ at a patient's actual blood temperature and attenuates the cerebral vasoconstriction caused by hypothermia. The use of pH stat during cooling may promote better cerebral protection through more homogenous and rapid brain cooling,[65] increased CBF,[66] and improved oxygen delivery due to higher flows and a rightward shift in the oxyhemoglobin dissociation curve. Although pH stat is not as well reported in the adult population, it may result in better postoperative outcomes.[2] In 182 infants undergoing cardiac surgery for congenital defects, the use of pH stat during cooling to deep HCA was associated with lower postoperative morbidity and a shorter recovery time to first EEG activity compared with an alpha stat strategy.[67] pH stat may also result in improved neurologic performance and less neuronal cell damage after undergoing deep HCA.[68] The authors' protocol requires pH stat to be continued during the circulatory arrest period to maintain a higher CBF and more evenly distributed oxygen supply to the brain. The use of pH stat during cerebral perfusion may significantly improve brain tissue blood flow and oxygenation.[69]

On rewarming, alpha stat management is used for the remainder of CPB. The utilization of alpha stat during the rewarming period may reduce the risk for cerebral emboli, edema, and hyperthermia relative to pH stat. In addition, the protocol requires that the arterial blood temperature be limited to 37°C, preventing cerebral hyperthermia.[70] Limiting arterial temperature to 37°C is best coupled with alpha stat to limit hyperthermic blood flow to the brain and to slow cerebral rewarming. Limiting the speed of rewarming may help to avoid a mismatch between oxygen supply and demand. In patients undergoing cardiac surgery, the percent decrease in jugular venous saturation during rewarming was significantly related to the rate of rewarming.[71] This effect was also documented in children undergoing cardiac operations where they were cooled to deep hypothermia. This study showed a significant correlation between the decrease in jugular venous oxygen saturation and rewarming rate.[72] If pH stat was used during this period, the brain might be at increased risk for ischemia due to a higher metabolic demand and embolic load.

The authors' acid-base management strategy for total arch repair attempts to use the benefits of alpha stat and pH stat at different stages during the procedure. pH stat may not offer any advantage while a patient is mildly hypothermic, so alpha stat is used to preserve intracellular buffering capacity and to allow a baseline assessment prior to transitioning to pH stat. pH stat is used during the cooling phase and circulatory arrest to promote homogenous cooling and a high level of oxygen delivery. Alpha stat is best used during rewarming to prevent cerebral hyperthermia, hypertension, edema, and to decrease the risk of emboli.

HEMATOCRIT

Blood hematocrit affects the efficacy of sACP and HCA. A higher hematocrit (25%–30% vs 10%–20%) has been shown to improve functional outcomes in animal studies, reduced intracranial pressure, improved perfusion pressures.[73,74]

REWARMING/CEREBRAL HYPERTHERMIA

Cerebral hyperthermia is a prevalent and underrecognized cause of neurologic injury in aortic surgery. Cerebral hyperthermia may be overlooked because stronger emphases can commonly, and perhaps mistakenly, be placed on intraoperative monitoring to detect brain desaturation and ischemia.[75] Cerebral hyperthermia maybe responsible for 50% to 80% of the neuropsychologic dysfunction seen after cardiac surgery.[76] The underlying mechanisms include exacerbation of ischemic injury, improved oxygen radical reduction, increased release of excitatory neurotransmitters (glutamine) to toxic levels, impaired recovery of energy metabolism, and enhanced inhibition of protein kinases.[77]

The brain is one of the most well perfused organs in the body. This blood supply and associated perfusion paradoxically make core brain temperature difficult to estimate clinically in the operating room based on temperature measurements used at less well perfused peripheral body sites. This difficulty in core brain temperature estimation and measurement is a focus on ongoing research and a contributor to the high incidence of hyperthermia in cardiac surgery. Stone and colleagues[78] compared cerebral temperature, measured using a direct cerebral probe, during HCA and rewarming to peripheral temperature monitors. The pulmonary artery was the most accurate site overall. The distal esophagus also is accurate in closed chest surgery, but this is not the case in aortic arch surgery. Distal esophageal temperature measurements may underestimate brain temperature as a result of the temperature loss from the open chest.[34] The nasopharynx is accurate during the cooling phase of CPB due to its close proximity to the brain and during sACP due to its shared blood supply via the external carotid artery.[78] During the rewarming phase, however, it may underestimate brain temperature by up to 4°C.[79] The tympanic membrane has similar accuracy to the nasopharynx but is slightly less accurate during rewarming. Bladder and rectal temperatures, although easily accessible, exhibit substantial lag behind cerebral temperatures.[78]

Rewarming a patient too quickly by increasing the oxygenator temperature to greater than or equal to 39°C, or attempting to completely rewarm the patient back to 38°C, results in cerebral hyperthermia. Fast rewarming in rats, including the strict avoidance of hyperthermia at the end of rewarming, has shown to increase histologic brain tissue damage and overall brain inflammation characterized by greater eosinophil infiltration and nuclear factor κB expression versus slow rewarming.[80] Slowing the rate of rewarming is effective at avoiding overwarming but is not without repercussions. Slow rewarming may prolong the duration of CPB and increase the risk of postoperative hypothermia. Grigore and colleagues[81] found that slowing the rewarming rate from 4°C to 6°C gradient between the CPB perfusate and nasopharyngeal monitor down to a less than 2°C gradient significantly improved postoperative cognitive performance. Continuous patient surface rewarming can prevent cerebral hyperthermia while minimizing postoperative periods of hypothermia.[82] Desaturation during rewarming of cerebral venous blood measured by jugular venous oxygen saturation less than 50% is associated with worse neurologic outcomes.[83] Kawahara and colleagues[84] found that slow rewarming reduced the episodes of cerebral desaturation and the overall duration of cerebral desaturation. These findings did not correlate, however, with a postoperative change in the Mini-Mental State Examination, a relatively insensitive neurologic test.

Prepared and expedient surgical planning to efficiently time the beginning of rewarming is essential.

SUMMARY

Neurologic injury is a potentially devastating complication of cardiac and aortic surgery. Surgical technique and perioperative care must diminish these risks. Current clinical practice and the underlying theories that neuroprotection is based on are derived from observational studies. Despite the lack of robust randomized trials, current evidence provides valid and clinically useful data. Innovative new technologies for intraoperative monitoring combined with evolving operative techniques will help direct circulatory management by identifying intraoperative and immediate postoperative conditions of cerebral and spinal cord ischemia. Future studies will evaluate both the efficacy of current techniques and the etiologies of neurologic injury to guide future neuroprotective interventions.

Perhaps the most important aspect of neuroprotection for aortic disease is regular surveillance of the disease when first diagnosed and subsequent preemptive aortic reconstruction when warranted. As the field of aortic surgery develops, stricter parameters for aortic disease resulting in repairs for complex aortic diseases will likely become the new standard.

REFERENCES

1. Dorotta I, Kimball-Jones P, Applegate R 2nd. Deep hypothermia and circulatory arrest in adults. Semin Cardiothorac Vasc Anesth 2007;11(1):66–76.
2. Svyatets M, Tolani K, Zhang M, et al. Perioperative management of deep hypothermic circulatory arrest. J Cardiothorac Vasc Anesth 2010;24(4):644–55.
3. Wilkey BJ, Weitzel NS. Anesthetic considerations for surgery on the aortic arch. Semin Cardiothorac Vasc Anesth 2016;20(4):265–72.
4. Stecker MM. Neurophysiology of surgical procedures for repair of the aortic arch. J Clin Neurophysiol 2007;24(4):310–5.
5. Stecker MM, Cheung AT, Pochettino A, et al. Deep hypothermic circulatory arrest: I. Effects of cooling on electroencephalogram and evoked potentials. Ann Thorac Surg 2001;71(1):14–21.
6. Stecker MM, Cheung AT, Pochettino A, et al. Deep hypothermic circulatory arrest: II. Changes in electroencephalogram and evoked potentials during rewarming. Ann Thorac Surg 2001;71(1):22–8.
7. James ML, Andersen ND, Swaminathan M, et al. Predictors of electrocerebral inactivity with deep hypothermia. J Thorac Cardiovasc Surg 2014;147(3): 1002–7.
8. Engelman R, Baker RA, Likosky DS, et al. The Society of Thoracic Surgeons, The Society of Cardiovascular Anesthesiologists, and The American Society of ExtraCorporeal Technology: Clinical practice guidelines for cardiopulmonary bypass–temperature management during cardiopulmonary bypass. Ann Thorac Surg 2015;100(2):748–57.
9. Mezrow CK, Midulla PS, Sadeghi AM, et al. Evaluation of cerebral metabolism and quantitative electroencephalography after hypothermic circulatory arrest and low-flow cardiopulmonary bypass at different temperatures. J Thorac Cardiovasc Surg 1994;107(4):1006–19.
10. Steppan J, Hogue CW Jr. Cerebral and tissue oximetry. Best Pract Res Clin Anaesthesiol 2014;28(4): 429–39.
11. Jobsis FF. Noninvasive, infrared monitoring of cerebral and myocardial oxygen sufficiency and circulatory parameters. Science 1977;198(4323):1264–7.
12. Zheng F, Sheinberg R, Yee MS, et al. Cerebral near-infrared spectroscopy monitoring and neurologic outcomes in adult cardiac surgery patients: a systematic review. Anesth Analg 2013;116(3):663–76.
13. Murkin JM. NIRS: a standard of care for CPB vs. an evolving standard for selective cerebral perfusion? J Extra Corpor Technol 2009;41(1):P11–4.
14. Olsson C, Thelin S. Regional cerebral saturation monitoring with near-infrared spectroscopy during selective antegrade cerebral perfusion: diagnostic performance and relationship to postoperative stroke. J Thorac Cardiovasc Surg 2006;131(2): 371–9.
15. Urbanski PP, Lenos A, Kolowca M, et al. Near-infrared spectroscopy for neuromonitoring of unilateral cerebral perfusion. Eur J Cardiothorac Surg 2013;43(6):1140–4.
16. Tobias JD, Russo P, Russo J. Changes in near infrared spectroscopy during deep hypothermic circulatory arrest. Ann Card Anaesth 2009;12(1):17–21.
17. Nollert G, Shin'oka T, Jonas RA. Near-infrared spectrophotometry of the brain in cardiovascular surgery. Thorac Cardiovasc Surg 1998;46(3):167–75.
18. Harrer M, Waldenberger FR, Weiss G, et al. Aortic arch surgery using bilateral antegrade selective cerebral perfusion in combination with near-infrared spectroscopy. Eur J Cardiothorac Surg 2010;38(5): 561–7.
19. Leyvi G, Bello R, Wasnick JD, et al. Assessment of cerebral oxygen balance during deep hypothermic circulatory arrest by continuous jugular bulb venous saturation and near-infrared spectroscopy. J Cardiothorac Vasc Anesth 2006;20(6):826–33.

20. Bavaria JE, Pochettino A, Brinster DR, et al. New paradigms and improved results for the surgical treatment of acute type A dissection. Ann Surg 2001;234(3):336–42 [discussion: 342–3].

21. Coselli JS, Crawford ES, Beall AC Jr, et al. Determination of brain temperatures for safe circulatory arrest during cardiovascular operation. Ann Thorac Surg 1988;45(6):638–42.

22. Svensson LG, Crawford ES, Hess KR, et al. Deep hypothermia with circulatory arrest. Determinants of stroke and early mortality in 656 patients. J Thorac Cardiovasc Surg 1993;106(1):19–28 [discussion 28–31].

23. Lima B, Williams JB, Bhattacharya SD, et al. Results of proximal arch replacement using deep hypothermia for circulatory arrest: is moderate hypothermia really justifiable? Am Surg 2011; 77(11):1438–44.

24. Svensson LG, Blackstone EH, Rajeswaran J, et al. Does the arterial cannulation site for circulatory arrest influence stroke risk? Ann Thorac Surg 2004; 78(4):1274–84 [discussion 1274–84].

25. Englum BR, Andersen ND, Husain AM, et al. Degree of hypothermia in aortic arch surgery - optimal temperature for cerebral and spinal protection: deep hypothermia remains the gold standard in the absence of randomized data. Ann Cardiothorac Surg 2013; 2(2):184–93.

26. Vallabhajosyula P, Jassar AS, Menon RS, et al. Moderate versus deep hypothermic circulatory arrest for elective aortic transverse hemiarch reconstruction. Ann Thorac Surg 2015;99(5):1511–7.

27. Tsai JY, Pan W, Lemaire SA, et al. Moderate hypothermia during aortic arch surgery is associated with reduced risk of early mortality. J Thorac Cardiovasc Surg 2013;146(3):662–7.

28. Kamiya H, Hagl C, Kropivnitskaya I, et al. The safety of moderate hypothermic lower body circulatory arrest with selective cerebral perfusion: a propensity score analysis. J Thorac Cardiovasc Surg 2007; 133(2):501–9.

29. Pacini D, Leone A, Di Marco L, et al. Antegrade selective cerebral perfusion in thoracic aorta surgery: safety of moderate hypothermia. Eur J Cardiothorac Surg 2007;31(4):618–22.

30. Leshnower BG, Myung RJ, Kilgo PD, et al. Moderate hypothermia and unilateral selective antegrade cerebral perfusion: a contemporary cerebral protection strategy for aortic arch surgery. Ann Thorac Surg 2010;90(2):547–54.

31. Livesay JJ, Cooley DA, Reul GJ, et al. Resection of aortic arch aneurysms: a comparison of hypothermic techniques in 60 patients. Ann Thorac Surg 1983;36(1):19–28.

32. Welz A, Pogarell O, Tatsch K, et al. Surgery of the thoracic aorta using deep hypothermic total circulatory arrest. Are there neurological consequences other than frank cerebral defects? Eur J Cardiothorac Surg 1997;11(4):650–6.

33. Angeloni E, Benedetto U, Takkenberg JJ, et al. Unilateral versus bilateral antegrade cerebral protection during circulatory arrest in aortic surgery: a meta-analysis of 5100 patients. J Thorac Cardiovasc Surg 2014;147(1):60–7.

34. Yan TD, Bannon PG, Bavaria J, et al. Consensus on hypothermia in aortic arch surgery. Ann Cardiothorac Surg 2013;2(2):163–8.

35. Keenan JE, Wang H, Ganapathi AM, et al. Electroencephalography during hemiarch replacement with moderate hypothermic circulatory arrest. Ann Thorac Surg 2016;101(2):631–7.

36. Ono M, Joshi B, Brady K, et al. Risks for impaired cerebral autoregulation during cardiopulmonary bypass and postoperative stroke. Br J Anaesth 2012;109(3):391–8.

37. Ono M, Brown C, Lee JK, et al. Cerebral blood flow autoregulation is preserved after hypothermic circulatory arrest. Ann Thorac Surg 2013;96(6):2045.

38. Reece TB, Tribble CG, Smith RL, et al. Central cannulation is safe in acute aortic dissection repair. J Thorac Cardiovasc Surg 2007;133(2):428–34.

39. Di Eusanio M, Pantaleo A, Petridis FD, et al. Impact of different cannulation strategies on in-hospital outcomes of aortic arch surgery: a propensity-score analysis. Ann Thorac Surg 2013;96(5):1656–63.

40. De Paulis R, Czerny M, Weltert L, et al. Current trends in cannulation and neuroprotection during surgery of the aortic arch in Europe. Eur J Cardiothorac Surg 2015;47(5):917–23.

41. Erbel R, Aboyans V, Boileau C, et al. 2014 ESC Guidelines on the diagnosis and treatment of aortic diseases: document covering acute and chronic aortic diseases of the thoracic and abdominal aorta of the adult. The Task Force for the Diagnosis and Treatment of Aortic Diseases of the European Society of Cardiology (ESC). Eur Heart J 2014;35(41):2873–926.

42. De Bakey ME, Crawford ES, Cooley DA, et al. Successful resection of fusiform aneurysm of aortic arch with replacement by homograft. Surg Gynecol Obstet 1957;105(6):657–64.

43. Jassar AS, Vallabhajosyula P, Bavaria JE, et al. Direct innominate artery cannulation: an alternate technique for antegrade cerebral perfusion during aortic hemiarch reconstruction. J Thorac Cardiovasc Surg 2016;151(4):1073–8.

44. Preventza O, Garcia A, Tuluca A, et al. Innominate artery cannulation for proximal aortic surgery: outcomes and neurological events in 263 patients. Eur J Cardiothorac Surg 2015;48(6):937–42 [discussion: 942].

45. Wong DR, Coselli JS, Palmero L, et al. Axillary artery cannulation in surgery for acute or subacute ascending aortic dissections. Ann Thorac Surg 2010;90(3):731–7.

46. Riggs HE, Rupp C. Variation in form of circle of Willis. The relation of the variations to collateral circulation: anatomic analysis. Arch Neurol 1963;8:8–14.

47. Orihashi K, Sueda T, Okada K, et al. Malposition of selective cerebral perfusion catheter is not a rare event. Eur J Cardiothorac Surg 2005;27(4):644–8.

48. Ehrlich MP, Hagl C, McCullough JN, et al. Retrograde cerebral perfusion provides negligible flow through brain capillaries in the pig. J Thorac Cardiovasc Surg 2001;122(2):331–8.

49. Boeckxstaens CJ, Flameng WJ. Retrograde cerebral perfusion does not perfuse the brain in nonhuman primates. Ann Thorac Surg 1995;60(2): 319–27 [discussion: 327–8].

50. Bonser RS, Wong CH, Harrington D, et al. Failure of retrograde cerebral perfusion to attenuate metabolic changes associated with hypothermic circulatory arrest. J Thorac Cardiovasc Surg 2002;123(5):943–50.

51. Harrington DK, Bonser M, Moss A, et al. Neuropsychometric outcome following aortic arch surgery: a prospective randomized trial of retrograde cerebral perfusion. J Thorac Cardiovasc Surg 2003;126(3): 638–44.

52. Wong KC. Physiology and pharmacology of hypothermia. West J Med 1983;138(2):227–32.

53. Griepp RB, Stinson EB, Hollingsworth JF, et al. Prosthetic replacement of the aortic arch. J Thorac Cardiovasc Surg 1975;70(6):1051–63.

54. Reich DL, Uysal S, Sliwinski M, et al. Neuropsychologic outcome after deep hypothermic circulatory arrest in adults. J Thorac Cardiovasc Surg 1999; 117(1):156–63.

55. Di Eusanio M, Wesselink RM, Morshuis WJ, et al. Deep hypothermic circulatory arrest and antegrade selective cerebral perfusion during ascending aorta-hemiarch replacement: a retrospective comparative study. J Thorac Cardiovasc Surg 2003;125(4):849–54.

56. McCullough JN, Zhang N, Reich DL, et al. Cerebral metabolic suppression during hypothermic circulatory arrest in humans. Ann Thorac Surg 1999; 67(6):1895–9 [discussion: 1919–21].

57. Westaby S. Coagulation disturbance in profound hypothermia: the influence of anti-fibrinolytic therapy. Semin Thorac Cardiovasc Surg 1997;9(3):246–56.

58. Alam HB, Duggan M, Li Y, et al. Putting life on hold-for how long? Profound hypothermic cardiopulmonary bypass in a Swine model of complex vascular injuries. J Trauma 2008;64(4):912–22.

59. O'Neill B, Bilal H, Mahmood S, et al. Is it worth packing the head with ice in patients undergoing deep hypothermic circulatory arrest? Interact Cardiovasc Thorac Surg 2012;15(4):696–701.

60. Zhurav L, Wildes TS. Pro: topical hypothermia should be used during deep hypothermic circulatory arrest. J Cardiothorac Vasc Anesth 2012;26(2): 333–6.

61. Grocott HP, Andreiw A. Con: topical head cooling should not be used during deep hypothermic circulatory arrest. J Cardiothorac Vasc Anesth 2012; 26(2):337–9.

62. Tinker JH. Cardiopulmonary bypass: current concepts and controversies. A Society of Cardiovascular Anesthesiologists monograph. Philadelphia: Saunders; 1989. p. x, 156.

63. Reeves RB. An imidazole alphastat hypothesis for vertebrate acid-base regulation: tissue carbon dioxide content and body temperature in bullfrogs. Respir Physiol 1972;14(1):219–36.

64. Li ZJ, Yin XM, Ye J. Effects of pH management during deep hypothermic bypass on cerebral oxygenation: alpha-stat versus pH-stat. J Zhejiang Univ Sci 2004;5(10):1290–7.

65. Kurth CD, O'Rourke MM, O'Hara IB. Comparison of pH-stat and alpha-stat cardiopulmonary bypass on cerebral oxygenation and blood flow in relation to hypothermic circulatory arrest in piglets. Anesthesiology 1998;89(1):110–8.

66. Schell RM, Kern FH, Greeley WJ, et al. Cerebral blood flow and metabolism during cardiopulmonary bypass. Anesth Analg 1993;76(4):849–65.

67. du Plessis AJ, Jonas RA, Wypij D, et al. Perioperative effects of alpha-stat versus pH-stat strategies for deep hypothermic cardiopulmonary bypass in infants. J Thorac Cardiovasc Surg 1997;114(6):991–1000 [discussion: 1000–1].

68. Priestley MA, Golden JA, O'Hara IB, et al. Comparison of neurologic outcome after deep hypothermic circulatory arrest with alpha-stat and pH-stat cardiopulmonary bypass in newborn pigs. J Thorac Cardiovasc Surg 2001;121(2):336–43.

69. Ye J, Li Z, Yang Y, et al. Use of a pH-stat strategy during retrograde cerebral perfusion improves cerebral perfusion and tissue oxygenation. Ann Thorac Surg 2004;77(5):1664–70 [discussion: 1670].

70. Shann KG, Likosky DS, Murkin JM, et al. An evidence-based review of the practice of cardiopulmonary bypass in adults: a focus on neurologic injury, glycemic control, hemodilution, and the inflammatory response. J Thorac Cardiovasc Surg 2006; 132(2):283–90.

71. Nakajima T, Kuro M, Hayashi Y, et al. Clinical evaluation of cerebral oxygen balance during cardiopulmonary bypass: on-line continuous monitoring of jugular venous oxyhemoglobin saturation. Anesth Analg 1992;74(5):630–5.

72. van der Linden J, Ekroth R, Lincoln C, et al. Is cerebral blood flow/metabolic mismatch during rewarming a risk factor after profound hypothermic procedures in small children? Eur J Cardiothorac Surg 1989;3(3):209–15.

73. Sakamoto T, Nollert GD, Zurakowski D, et al. Hemodilution elevates cerebral blood flow and oxygen metabolism during cardiopulmonary bypass in

piglets. Ann Thorac Surg 2004;77(5):1656–63 [discussion: 1663].

74. Halstead JC, Wurm M, Meier DM, et al. Avoidance of hemodilution during selective cerebral perfusion enhances neurobehavioral outcome in a survival porcine model. Eur J Cardiothorac Surg 2007; 32(3):514–20.

75. Campos JM, Paniagua P. Hypothermia during cardiac surgery. Best Pract Res Clin Anaesthesiol 2008;22(4):695–709.

76. Engelman RM, Pleet AB, Rousou JA, et al. Influence of cardiopulmonary bypass perfusion temperature on neurologic and hematologic function after coronary artery bypass grafting. Ann Thorac Surg 1999;67(6):1547–55 [discussion: 1556].

77. Ginsberg MD, Busto R. Combating hyperthermia in acute stroke: a significant clinical concern. Stroke 1998;29(2):529–34.

78. Stone JG, Young WL, Smith CR, et al. Do standard monitoring sites reflect true brain temperature when profound hypothermia is rapidly induced and reversed? Anesthesiology 1995;82(2):344–51.

79. Kaukuntla H, Harrington D, Bilkoo I, et al. Temperature monitoring during cardiopulmonary bypass–do we undercool or overheat the brain? Eur J Cardiothorac Surg 2004;26(3):580–5.

80. Gordan ML, Kellermann K, Blobner M, et al. Fast rewarming after deep hypothermic circulatory arrest in rats impairs histologic outcome and increases NFkappaB expression in the brain. Perfusion 2010; 25(5):349–54.

81. Grigore AM, Grocott HP, Mathew JP, et al. The rewarming rate and increased peak temperature alter neurocognitive outcome after cardiac surgery. Anesth Analg 2002;94(1):4–10. table of contents.

82. Bar-Yosef S, Mathew JP, Newman MF, et al. Prevention of cerebral hyperthermia during cardiac surgery by limiting on-bypass rewarming in combination with post-bypass body surface warming: a feasibility study. Anesth Analg 2004;99(3):641–6. table of contents.

83. Croughwell ND, Newman MF, Blumenthal JA, et al. Jugular bulb saturation and cognitive dysfunction after cardiopulmonary bypass. Ann Thorac Surg 1994; 58(6):1702–8.

84. Kawahara F, Kadoi Y, Saito S, et al. Slow rewarming improves jugular venous oxygen saturation during rewarming. Acta Anaesthesiol Scand 2003;47(4): 419–24.

Moving?

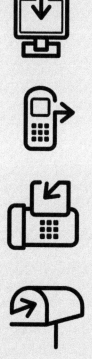

Printed and bound by CPI Group (UK) Ltd, Croydon, CR0 4YY

03/10/2024

01040302-0014